A HISTORY OF
WAR
SURGERY

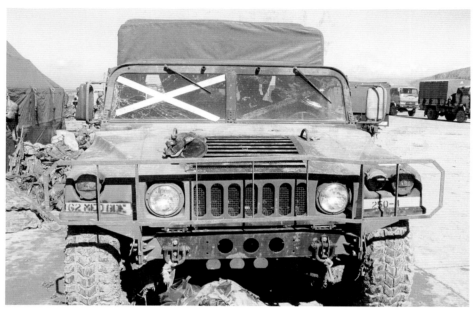

A humvee just landed by parachute with other components of a Forward Surgical Team (FST) assembled nearby. (*Dr G. Peoples*)

A HISTORY OF
WAR
SURGERY

DR JOHN WRIGHT

AMBERLEY

To Mary Hanigan who taught me to read, and to those who sacrifice in war and those who would mend them.

First published 2011

Amberley Publishing
The Hill, Stroud,
Gloucestershire, GL5 4ER

www.amberleybooks.com

Copyright © Dr John Wright 2011

British Library Cataloguing in Publication Data.
A catalogue record for this book is available from the British Library.

ISBN 978-1-4456-0232-5

Typesetting and Origination by Amberley Publishing.
Printed in Great Britain.

Contents

Acknowledgements

Many illustrations and references in this book were provided by United States and Australian military and memorial sources, among others.

I am deeply indebted to the following in particular: Australian Department of Defence; Australian War Memorial, Canberra; British War Memorial, London; Department of Veterans' Affairs, Canberra; Department of Defence, USA; International Red Cross (IRC); Marine Corps Archives, USA; Médecins Sans Frontières (MSF); National Archives and Records Administration, USA; National Library of Medicine, USA; Navy Yard, Washington, USA; US Army Medical Department and Public Affairs; US Army Surgeon General's Department.

Every effort has been made to locate the copyright holders of photographs and illustrations where the source was uncertain.

Without assistance from the following, this story could not have been told. I am profoundly grateful to them: Clive Baker, Dr Greg Bruce, Karen Brulliard (*Washington Post*), Marian Chirichella (WRAMC), Dr Michael Crumplin, Dr Michael E. DeBakey, Dr Michael Echols, Edwin Finney, Arnold Freeman, John Gibbins, Dr Richard Gordon, John Greenwood, Dr Ron Hoy, Phillip Knightley, Andreea Mills, Harry Noyes, Dr George Peoples, Rob Ruggenberg, Colonel Peter Sharwood, Colonel Harry Stinger, James K. Sunshine, Laura Waayers.

Christina Litchfield's secretarial expertise was meticulous and generous at all times; Irina Dunn's literary experience made all things possible; and Amberley's superlative publishing experience and encouragement were indispensable and enduring.

The endless encouragement, advice and patience of my wife, Rebecca, made the whole enterprise feasible and worthwhile.

Foreword

If aliens from outer space ever visit our earth, one aspect of our behaviour will certainly bewilder them. Why does one group of earthlings devote so much time and energy to trying to destroy another? Why do men bomb, shoot, kill and maim their fellow creatures and then watch as others of the same species devote their time and skill to trying to put them together again.

The extra-terrestrials will reach the same conclusion as John Wright has in this comprehensive, important, ground-breaking book: it is illogical; it makes no sense and it is indefensible. Dr Wright is not interested in writing about the first group, the men who do the damage. He is fascinated by the second, the war surgeons who throughout history have done their best to save the lives of men torn apart by the ever-increasing sophistication of weapons of war.

The arms manufacturers have shown diabolical skill and ingenuity in their work, devising weapons deliberately designed to inflict maximum damage to the human body, then retreating a step so that a soldier is maimed, not killed outright. The calculation is that the cost and time of long-term care is a more efficient drain on resources than an outright kill. The manufacturers of cluster bombs, those small but deadly explosive devices that air forces scatter around war zones like confetti, design them in bright colours to attract children's attention.

It was not always so. Dr Wright's history shows how the Greeks and Romans largely confined their armies to professional soldiers and looked after their wounded with skill and dedication. The war surgeons of the day knew how to 'cut out darts and relieve the smarting of wounds ... raise the dead and rank as God ... delivering [those] wounded by bronze or far-flung stones ... with herbal cures or with his knife'. Dr Wright takes us on a gripping tour of battlefields over the centuries and explains the slow evolution of the skills needed to save lives, from treating gunpowder wounds with boiling oil in the sixteenth century, to amputations without anaesthetic in the eighteenth and the high-tech operating theatres dealing with the victims of the Iraq War in the twenty-first.

This is not a book for the squeamish. It is heavily illustrated with graphic photographs of war surgeons at work; it tells us how war surgeons see their profession, how they feel about it and, above all, how they regard a society that makes what they do so necessary but, unless we change our ways, ultimately so futile.

Phillip Knightley, London, 2009

Preface

It is the soldier, not the poet, who gives us freedom of speech. It is the soldier, not the reporter, who gives us freedom of the press. It is the soldier, not the camp organiser, who gives us freedom to protest. It is the soldier who serves beneath the flag, salutes the flag and whose coffin is draped by the flag, who gives us the right to burn the flag.

– Padre D. E. O'Brien, US Marine Corps, Reunion Day, 1990

When the distinguished author and my friend from schooldays Phillip Knightley suggested a few years ago that I should write something about war surgery, I began to wonder what those surgeons and their gallant teams actually did and felt at work. What drove them? What were their fears, joys and regrets? As I delved further into this intriguing subject, I realised that little was known about the fascinating history of war surgery, and decided to accept Phillip's advice to write a book about it.

Phillip and I were born in Sydney between the great world wars. Returned soldiers from the First World War or 'legacy children'[1] wore their badges proudly; some men were disfigured by scars and those who had not lost legs still walked differently from other men. Even the remote dominion of Australia had quaked as it became a Japanese target in the Second World War.

Just as we were finishing school and our parents were fearing that yet another son from our street might have to wear a uniform and perhaps die, the war ended. When the men and women who had survived came home, our teenage eyes watched a new crop of old 'Diggers' bear the scars of war as they marched along George Street on Anzac Day.

Ten years later, Phillip was establishing his illustrious career in London and I had graduated in Medicine in Sydney. I began serious operating in the earliest days of open-heart and cancer surgery, when most of what we know now was waiting to be learned.

---

1. 'Legacy' is an Australian organisation established in 1923 to help support widows and children of lost servicemen.

My research for this book suggests that war surgery resembles the 'hell-and-high-water' years of my own experience some fifty years ago. Fear of, and frustration and anger at our limitations filled the professional lives of us surgeons. Medicines rarely helped. Heart diseases that can be safely corrected today were death sentences then. Surgery on blood vessels was fraught with risks of torrential haemorrhage. Psychiatric disorders were treated by isolation in places more like prisons than hospitals. New antibiotics were slow to emerge after penicillin. Scans were still twenty years away, heroin was freely prescribed with Latin symbols, and intensive care wards were still to develop. War surgery changed all of that inertia.

Detailed information about war surgeons, their colleagues and the places where they worked could be learned from personal stories, from the mass media, and from recorded history. These sources govern the scope of my enquiry. For closer examination of today's conflicts, it is virtually impossible (and extremely dangerous) to visit any of those areas unless sponsored by a reputable media organisation or embedded within a formal army. Neither of these options are feasible or acceptable if one's motive is to write about how wars really work. Even 'official' correspondents are rarely allowed beyond the protected 'green zones' to see surgical teams at work on the worst human casualties.

However, this is not a history of warfare. Countless publications by individuals and governments have done that expertly in great detail. My sole purpose has been to examine what all types of medical people and their patients must experience in combat, and how that experience has developed and changed over the centuries. My primary wish has been to understand the challenges that faced war surgeons and their teams, how they responded to those challenges, and how successful they were in overcoming seemingly insurmountable obstacles in extraordinarily difficult conditions.

I have examined many reports and scenes of combat surgery, much of it in remote, primitive places, and I have spoken to, or corresponded with, surgeons, soldiers, medics and technicians who have served in wars. I feared there might be a natural reluctance to relive perilous days, but I was received with great warmth by my interviewees. I expected that time had blunted some of the deadly urgency of those momentous events, and I knew that the memories of some participants may be unreliable in their detail. Even primary sources do not always agree on details of incidents and battles that are morbid, terrifying and confusing.

Despite their limitations, I have relied particularly on the scarce, first-hand verbal and written accounts of the carers and the cared for, especially those recorded closely to the events experienced. Wherever possible, I have included verbatim statements by those who were actually 'there'. They depict stark events and visceral responses that most of us have never known or thought much about. From these, I have collected fragments of the awful conditions of war and the selfless contributions of medical people who work with what nobody else can confront or begin to repair.

The period of war surgery that might be considered in some way 'scientific' is that of the last century. The more wars we have, the better we get at all types of surgery. They have taught surgeons how to manage catastrophic injuries and states of shock. Rapid transportation and evacuation systems save countless lives that were once doomed. We have learned how to frustrate the germs of gas gangrene and tetanus, to use antibiotics generally, to understand cold injury, blood transfusion, blast injuries, the effects of terrorism on communities and individuals, and how nutrition, hygiene and morale make armies work and win more effectively. We now know a great deal about 'shell-shock', that elusive thief of minds. All of these prizes have overflowed directly from wars to civilian life, but we have still not learned to control the manufacture and distribution of arms to anybody who can afford them, or how to protect the most vulnerable of humanity from them.

Salvaging something good from the terrible violence of battlefields is the province of special people – surgeons, anaesthetists, nurses, medics, stretcher-bearers, rescue and helicopter crews, bomb disposal experts, technicians and many others who work close to the action. Whatever their reasons for being there, surgical teams choose to deal with the appalling results of wars, and in doing so they derive one of the greatest and most primitive elements of human gratification: the identification and restoration of what is damaged.

However, under the pressure of warfare, where the principles of triage are 'to fix what you can and to avoid futile treatment for those you cannot help', many surgeons have faced ethical conflicts that challenge their allegiance to the Hippocratic oath. The ways in which these conflicts have been dealt with is a fascinating study in itself.

This book is an unqualified tribute to the unique dedication and generosity of doctors and their teams who try to make something good out of awful tragedy. I have tried to tell their story and present an account of their work that gives readers a chance to learn about this unfairly neglected but uniquely interesting field of medical, military and, indeed, social history.

John Wright

Medical and Military Time Line
AD 1–2009

476	Collapse of the Western Roman Empire and start of the Middle Ages
765	Baghdad Medical School founded
900	Gunpowder first described
1180	First French medical school founded at Montpellier
1337–1453	Hundred Years War
1300s	Start of the Renaissance; doctors and surgeons first 'qualified'
1424	Master Surgeons' Guild established in London
1530	Opium analgesia introduced into Europe
1540	Ether discovered; Union of Barber Surgeons and Physicians, London, tentatively agreed; germ particle theory proposed
1543	Vesalius writes first textbook and atlas on anatomy, Belgium
1572	Paré writes on gunshot wounds and antiseptics
1628	Harvey discovers blood circulation; first attempted blood transfusion
1745	Company of Surgeons separates from Barbers
1766–1842	Life of Baron Larrey, Napoleon's favourite battle surgeon, famous for insisting upon the rapid evacuation of the wounded
1775–83	American War of Independence
1790–1800	Ether, chloroform and nitrous oxide first used as general anaesthetics in battle surgery; Jenner discovers vaccination; accurate rifles developed from clumsy muskets
1800	Establishment of the exclusive Royal College of Surgeons in England
1803	The extraction of morphine from opium is pioneered by Friedrich Serturner in Germany
1805	Battle of Trafalgar; death of Horatio Nelson
1815	Battle of Waterloo
1815	Curare from South America adapted by Brody to aid muscle relaxation for deep surgery
1842–46	General anaesthesia developed and refined
1847	Sommeliers show germs in disease transmission
1848	Adhesive tape invented
1853	Injecting syringe developed

1854	Crimean War
1858	Gray's Anatomy textbook first published
1860	Florence Nightingale School of nursing founded in London
1861	Pasteur identifies bacteria
1863	Red Cross founded, Geneva
1861–65	American Civil War
1865	Lister uses carbolic acid as antiseptic
1870	Koch extends Lister's work with bacteria
1890	Surgical gloves manufactured by Halsted
1895	X-rays discovered by Roentgen
1899–1902	Boer War
1905	First blood transfusion from donor artery to patient vein performed by George Crile
1908	Sulpha drugs synthesised
1913	American College of Surgeons founded
1914	Archibald conducts the first, now conventional, transfusion of stored blood
1914–18	The First World War
1922	Mussolini becomes Prime Minister of Italy
1925	The structural formula of morphine is determined by Janos Kabay in Hungary, allowing its synthesis
1928	Fleming discovers penicillin
1933	Hitler becomes German Chancellor; sulphonamide patented
1936–39	Spanish Civil War
1939–45	The Second World War
1940	Florey extends penicillin use
1950–53	Korean War
1960–73	Vietnam War
1980–88	Iran/Iraq War
1981–82	Falklands War
1989	Cold War ends
1990–91	Gulf War (Desert Storm)
2000	Sub-Saharan wars escalate
2001	Afghan War begins; 9/11 attack on New York's World Trade Center
2003	Iraq War begins
2002	Bali bombing
2003	Iraq Freedom War; Darfur, Sudan War
2004	Madrid bombing
2005	London bombing
2006	Israel/Hezbollah War; Mumbai bombing
2007	First North Korea nuclear test; Israel/Palestine conflict intensifies
2009	North Korea nuclear tests
2009	Pakistan bombings and the Afghan War escalates

CHAPTER 1

Evolution of War Surgery

In the midst of peace, Roman troops familiarised themselves with the practice of war; and it is prettily remarked by an ancient historian who had fought against them, that the effusion of blood was the only circumstance which distinguished the field of battle from the field of exercise.

– Edward Gibbon, *The Decline and Fall of the Roman Empire*, 1794

One surgeon is worth an army of men.

– Homer, *The Iliad*, XI, 700 BC

Human skulls displaying evidence of surgical operations from 15,000 years ago have been found in burial sites in Europe, Egypt and South America. Some operations were for caved-in fractures sustained in fights or accidents, while others had probably been carried out to treat psychiatric disorders, intractable headaches, epilepsy, tumours and spiritual uncertainties.

Egyptian surgeons were the first to persuade soldiers to wear helmets in war. They knew that the removal of dead tissue and debris from wounds (later called 'debridement' by the French, but known by many other names such as 'epluchage', or peeling, and 'parage', or paring) was fundamental to the safe healing of wounds. They saw that these measures were effective, just as they saw that psychotherapy helped to calm frightened soldiers. In 1862, ancient surgical history became much clearer when Edwin Smith, an American Egyptologist, discovered a 5,000-year-old surgical text on human anatomy and the surgery of injuries.

In 400 BC, the great Greek physician Hippocrates realised that above all other teaching methods, surgeons needed wars to extend their skills:

He who wants to be a skilful surgeon must have sufficient experience of military surgery, namely, war surgery. Therefore he has to be drafted in foreign mercenary armies, and follow them in the field of battle, in order to operate on war wounds, to remove missiles and foreign bodies, and only thus may he have a full surgical education and a complete technical dexterity.

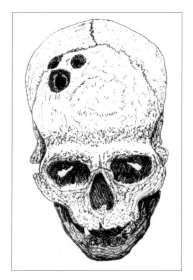

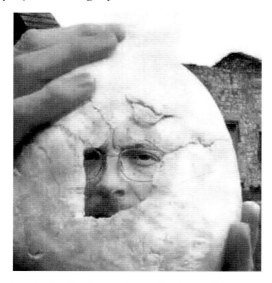

Above left: French skull with skilful trephine holes for inspection and release of distress, from about 8000 BC. (*Wikipedia*)

Above right: A trephined skull from about 960 BC found in England. Smooth, well-healed bone edges show the patient survived for years after surgery. (*Origin unknown*)

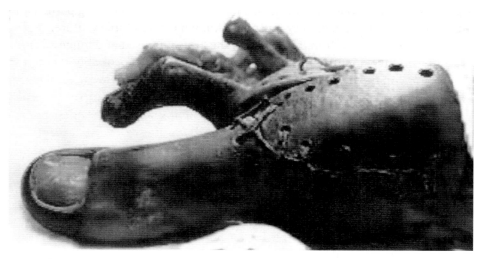

A prosthetic toe (probable a replacement for loss in battle) dating from 200 BC, made of wood and leather, and found in Egypt. (*Wikipedia*)

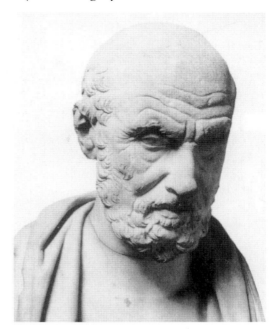

Hippocrates, father of modern medicine, born 460 BC. His teachings have been accepted by all Western doctors.

Perhaps as a result, in AD 100 enterprising Arabic surgeons confidently stitched the leg of a dead soldier onto the stump of a living amputee. All surviving participants were bitterly disappointed. They must have known it was a futile venture.

Without doubt, the Roman Army was the best organised and longest lasting western military institution in the ancient world. It was probably the first to formally recognise that, alongside regular army surgeons, veterinary surgeons were an integral part of an army that relied on animals for battle, transport and communication. In the Roman world, surgeons were ultimately responsible for the medical practices of both civilian and military life. They wrote the first western textbook of surgery in about AD 1200; it shows that they firmly believed in the need for cleanliness, even if they had no idea of how or why it reduced infection and death from surgical procedures; they certainly knew that quick amputation could abort gangrene in dirty wounds. Their forts and camps were built away from swamps that bred mosquitoes carrying malaria and other fevers. In addition, they built the first isolation hospitals for infected patients and they installed central heating.

Greek surgeons learned much from the Romans and repaid them by helping with Roman military and medical planning. Clearly, they were physicians who also knew how to perform complicated surgery. They saw themselves as:

… [knowing] … how to cut out darts and relieve the smarting of wounds … able to raise the dead and rank as a God … delivering [those] wounded by bronze or far-flung stones … with herbal cures … or with his knife.

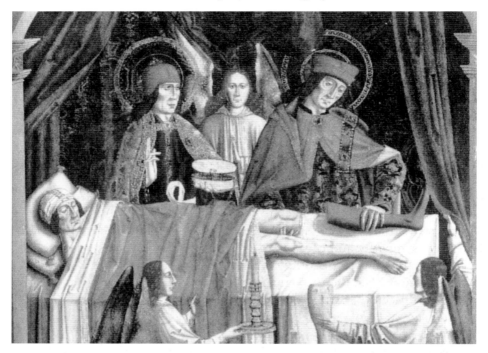

A medieval artist's impression of 'saints-at-surgery'. Note the interracial transplantation with no chance of success. (*Richard Gordon*)

Sadly, it was a thousand years before the rest of Europe caught up to the level reached by Roman medicine when the Empire fell.

* * *

The Renaissance did not only bring cultural and artistic advances, but also gunpowder, which enabled military commanders to inflict much more devastating injuries on men than had ever been seen before. It was when Paré, a celebrated French surgeon of the sixteenth century, was able to write about gunshot wounds and ligatures. He was also sure that a broth of eggs, oil of roses and turpentine was much superior to boiling oil in the treatment of gunpowder wounds, but that passing fantasy saved no lives and was soon forgotten. Happily, his troops considered him worth 10,000 foot soldiers because they believed that their chances of survival were greater from his mere presence on the battlefield.

In the mid-nineteenth century, much more complicated and prolonged surgical procedures became possible when ether and chloroform anaesthesia were first introduced into operating rooms. For the first time, men were able to tolerate intensive surgery while deeply asleep, pain-free and motionless. Before long, Semmelweis, Pasteur, Lister and Koch revolutionised surgical history by showing that infection was produced by germs called 'bacteria' – a focus for surgical study was at last available.

Lister was so impressed with the value of carbolic acid (Phenol of today) in killing germs within surgical wounds that he proudly announced to the world in 1866 that he had discovered 'one of the ten most important things that ever happened to the human race'. Certainly, the numbers of military amputations for gangrenous infections began to fall for the first time in history.

As Hippocrates said, if there is anything good at all about wars, it is that they accelerate medical and surgical advances; they are crash-courses in trauma for medical workers. The Greeks called surgery 'the manual manipulation carried out by the surgical practitioner to assuage the injuries and diseases of his or her fellows'. Its roots stretch back to the origins of humanity when surgeons and priests vied for the provision of physical and spiritual welfare to soldiers. Both gave sympathy and comfort to the wounded and dying, and attended to wounds. Priests used the titles of chaplain or padre and wore the cloth of their profession when they accompanied the Crusades. Appearance as well as expertise apparently mattered to Frederick the Great, who insisted that his surgeons should be 'of good repute, learned and, if possible, still wearing their own hair'.

At Waterloo, there was but one chaplain for every British Army division. Napoleon's Army had none. Instead, military academies in Europe were intent on imparting heroic, Christian qualities to their graduates, regardless of their talent for war. They were seen as potential officers of God rather than soldiers and leaders, and some, with no medical training at all, turned to surgery. The results were disastrous, but their God allowed them to kill men while under his personal protection. How that was reconciled with an enemy enjoying identical religious shelter has remained a matter for speculation.

MEDICAL POLITICS AT WORK

Rivalry between 'physicians' and 'surgeons' was forged thousands of years ago when the treatment of physical injuries clearly divided medical practitioners into two groups – those who were prepared to perform surgical operations, even if untrained, and those who were not. It was largely a matter of personal predisposition. Physicians specialised in secret, herbal tonics and regarded themselves as better educated than surgeons. They cured nobody, but rarely did positive harm, except by neglect. If one of their patients died, it was impossible to blame the treatment when everybody knew that most patients with serious illnesses died anyway, regardless of treatment.

Unfortunately for them, surgeons' interventions had obvious effects on the health of their patients. Major surgery on sick people carried an enormous risk and the surgeon could always be blamed. Indeed, there were surgical malpractice lawsuits in England in the fourteenth century. But with increasing recognition of their unique capabilities, surgeons were becoming the best paid and the most highly respected medical practitioners in the land. As well as having a deep understanding of 'real' information like anatomy, physiology and pathology, they were seen as men of stamina and ingenuity – even miracle-workers.

Oddly enough, in a description of 'doctors' of the fourteenth century, Chaucer never once mentioned the performance of surgical procedures. Maybe he regarded them as trivial. Physicians still saw themselves as intellectuals who actually 'understood' things. It was as if they had secret 'intellectual property' guiding them. They believed that they 'owned' pieces of medical knowledge, which gave them a uniquely 'learned' character. By those lofty standards, surgeons were merely craftsmen – such crude technicians that even barbers, priests and academy cadets could perform surgery if they felt inclined.

By the end of the Middle Ages, three distinctly different sorts of practitioners had evolved: 'physicians', who dealt with 'malformations and disorders of the

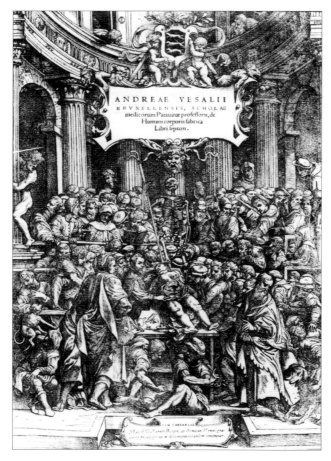

Vesalius (centre left), born in Belgium in 1514, was a pioneering teacher of anatomy.
(*Richard Gordon*)

complexion' (whatever those were!); 'surgeons', dealing with trauma, war wounds and major diseases the physicians could not and did not want to treat; and barbers, performing minor surgery, often in war. But just when surgeons were beginning to develop a superior image, the Church suddenly decreed that surgery was 'unclean and Godless' – studies of anatomy, experimentation with blood transfusion, draining of abscesses, surgical operations and vaccinations were outlawed.

It took a few hundred years of surgically neglected priests, soldiers and bureaucrats, and much clandestine scheming, for the blessing and support of the Church to be reinstated with the creation of a joint medical and surgical college at the end of the fourteenth century. The constant fighting of wars had come to persuade the Church that medicine was no less academic and practical a pursuit than theology or law. When the surgical 'guilds' affiliated themselves with British universities and created six-year courses of training and a certification process, surgery could never be challenged again. Churchmen were soon to become the surgeons' greatest admirers and most grateful patients.

Four hundred years later, the 'Company of Surgeons' separated entirely from the 'barbers' and established an independent professional body having equal stature to the physicians' colleges. The Royal College of Surgeons of England was established in 1800 and convinced its Fellows that they were completely legitimate 'physicians who specialised in surgery'. There was no subtlety in that description. It was meant to show once and for all that physicians had no answers to the conditions that surgeons treated.

WHAT A DIFFERENCE A WAR MAKES

War focussed the attention of military and political leaders on finding something better than leeches, salves, purges, potions and 'masterly inactivity' for the treatment of serious illness or injury. By the beginning of the sixteenth century, surgeons had become essential to armies, precipitating the end of knights and untrained soldiers practising medicine in battle.

The British had twenty surgeons at Agincourt to care for the sick and wounded, but they were scarcely needed when the battle turned into a blood-bath for the French, who were slaughtered by British arrows. The enormous numbers of wounded could not be evacuated and surgical help was not expected by the French troops who then knew little or nothing of the value of war surgery.

Perhaps the most powerful stimulus for military surgery came from spectacular events that would never be forgotten by historians. In AD 1199, Richard I of England suffered a serious arrow wound to his arm. Unfortunately, his personal physician had just retired from the army and returned to England to become Bishop of Worcester. With no one else on hand, one of Richard's mercenaries, who promoted himself as a medical practitioner though he was completely unqualified, confidently offered to treat the injury.

With no general anaesthesia or special instruments, he undertook a prolonged and gruesome intervention, and even then failed to extract the arrow. Richard almost certainly had a gangrenous infection of the shredded wound; within a few days, the King was dead. But, in a military sense, the mercenary's contribution was great – the value of the military surgeon had been emphasised as never before. Who could ever again run a war successfully without surgeons?

Centuries later, on the same side of the English Channel, Napoleon was much more fortunate. At Toulon in 1793, he suffered three significant injuries, two of them by bayonet and the other from a fall from his horse. During his active military career, twenty horses had fallen beneath him from accidents or injuries as he rode, but he survived all those hazards and fought on. It was suggested that his agonising haemorrhoids and urethral stricture, causing him to ride crookedly in the saddle, was to blame for his bad luck, but his personal valet hotly denied that theory.

A particularly gruesome incident occurred in 1814 when Napoleon rode directly across an exploding shell. It disembowelled his horse, causing it to fall heavily, but once again, Napoleon survived without a scratch for his surgeon to treat. For all ailments and incidents he was treated exclusively and successfully by his favourite, Baron Dominique Jean Larrey, whose surgical reputation rose to great heights and remained strong after his death.

It may come as a surprise that a benign rivalry between surgeons and physicians continues today, based on their own perceptions of their particular prerogatives, medico-political power and economic status. While there may be some differences in concepts of treatment, there is no argument at all about treating the injuries of war – surgeons have that all to themselves. With the challenges imposed by civilian trauma and the proliferating weapons of warfare and terrorism, the unique position of surgeons has become increasingly obvious. Like stretcher-bearers, helicopter pilots and medics, war surgeons are non-combatants who endure great personal risks to salvage injured soldiers quickly enough to return them to battle capability or fitness for civilian life.

GUNSHOT, GERMS AND GENTLEMEN

The introduction of gunpowder to war during the seventeenth and eighteenth centuries changed battle injuries forever. Hand-guns, muskets, cannon and rifles were the new instruments of devastation; the worst of it couldn't be fixed by any surgical techniques of the time. An English surgeon at the Battle of Waterloo made depressing notes about his workplace:

It is impossible to convey to you the picture of human misery continually before my eyes – while I amputated one man's thigh, there lay at one time thirteen others, all beseeching to be taken next – it was a strange thing to feel my clothes stiff with blood and my arms powerless from the exertion of using the knife. The gallant sorties, the charges, the individual instances of enterprise and valour before me, gave the sense that the world has had a victory at Waterloo. But that is a transient sense of victory, a gloomy uncomfortable view of human nature, the inevitable consequence of looking upon the whole as I did.

In 1847, Ignaz Semmelweis, a German-Hungarian physician in Vienna, had discovered that the deadly obstetric infection called 'child-bed fever' was being spread by doctors who delivered babies without bothering to wash their hands. Pasteur from France and Koch from Germany already knew about bacteria and, on the back of these giants of bacteriology, medical research was to take a giant leap. Army surgeons had realised that wound infection and gangrene came from the germs seething in manured battlefields, but military

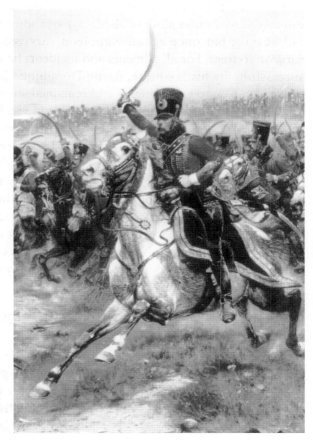

Curved swords inflicted deep and usually fatal lacerations at Waterloo. (*NSW Art Gallery, Sydney*)

commanders had no time for esoteric details; they sought military supremacy at any cost, and many of them belittled new medical discoveries that promised to save countless lives.

Britain had traditionally drawn its permanent army officers and surgeons from the 'gentlemen' of society, but whatever they had once been, inactivity between Waterloo and the First World War had rendered them out of touch with modern military and surgical practice. The Crimean War was a prime example: as well as being a military disaster, only moderately relieved by the influence of Florence Nightingale and her collaborators, it did little to enhance the reputation of surgeons at large. Their innovations had stalled simply because there was no stimulus to 'learn new tricks', having been involved in only one major European war for a century before Crimea.

It is difficult to believe a single day's conflict in the Napoleonic Wars could have resulted in many more military and civilian losses (counting French, Russian, Prussian, Austrian, Spanish, German, Polish and British casualties from wounds, infections, diseases, starvation, exposure, drowning, friendly fire, atrocities and other causes) than many South Pacific campaigns in the Second World War, for example, or than the entire US losses (58,000) in Vietnam. The credit for a precipitous fall in military death rates in the late-nineteenth century lies primarily with surgeons. They recognised that an army at war constituted a vast teaching laboratory of surgical and medical research. Physicians could only stand by and admire the ingenuity and courage of surgeons as they hastily exploited the ingenious discoveries of bacteriologists, immunologists and chemists.

As the First World War advanced, even the complicated injuries of vastly more damaging new missiles, aircraft and incendiary devices became more manageable with the help of the sulphonamides and, even better, penicillin. Above all else, surgeons repeatedly showed that innovation, improvisation and skill in wound management, particularly if contaminated, were essential if wars were to be won at prices worth paying.

THE WATERLOO EXPERIENCE

In a scholarly analysis of the Napoleonic Wars of 200 years ago, Michael Crumplin, surgeon and military historian, observed that those twenty-two years of conflict had been, in fact, the first 'world' war. In these wars, the greatest cause of death was still disease rather than injury; surgeons were hampered by their ignorance of the causes of infection, a lack of competent nurses and a total absence of general anaesthesia. British Army surgeons were in short supply and campaigns were often conducted in extreme climatic conditions.

To make matters worse, the central army bureaucracy was ignorant and unsympathetic. Senior officers insisted on being treated first and too few nurses meant that cooks, soldiers' wives and camp followers were called on for assistance. The ancient medical principles of the Romans – the importance of military teaching, veterinary surgeons for horses, cleanliness, organisation, training, rapid evacuation of wounded, avoidance of insect infestation, early amputation to avoid gangrene and isolation techniques to prevent cross-infection – had been long forgotten. At Waterloo, the British Army relied on 1,500 untrained and frightened soldiers to act as medics, stretcher-bearers and combat surgeons – with disastrous results. Surgeons had to provide their own mules to carry bags of instruments, water bottles, splints, dressings and tourniquets. There is little argument that the French surgeons, Larrey and Percy, had given their army superiority over the stodgy British, especially with their celebrated 'flying ambulances', which not only enabled more rapid evacuation of injured troops from the battle front, but also carried surgeons, assistants, supplies and stretcher-bearers more quickly into action.

Surgeons operated in all weather in their shirt sleeves, boots and an apron. With no notion of sterility, they used the same filthy rags to clean their tables, instruments, hands and arms, as they did to wash out patients' wounds. Without general anaesthesia, they were fully occupied with amputations, wrenching-out deeply embedded shrapnel, opening skulls to remove blood clots, blood-letting and the splinting of fractures.

Serious head, chest and abdominal injuries defied all surgical treatment. Any major amputation killed one man in four, even if it was done soon after injury.

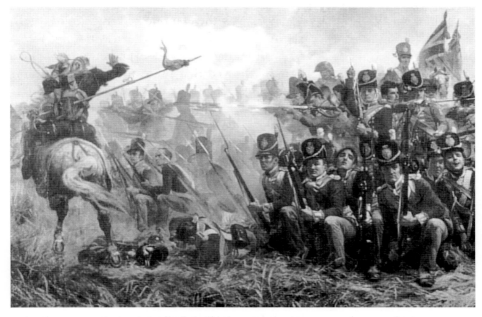

A painting of a scene in the Battle of Waterloo with multiple weapon types, cavalry and close-quarter infantry fighting. (*NSW Art Gallery, Sydney*)

If infection had already developed, almost all of them died. No matter who did the surgery and where, those deadly statistics didn't improve for a hundred years. Worst of all, there was very little understanding of the management of pain, and analgesic drugs were in short supply.

There were leg prostheses available, but there was none for arms. While carpenters occasionally made a rough 'peg-leg' for the common soldier, wealthy amputees could have a wooden leg tailor-made to their specifications. The Earl of Uxbridge, who lost a leg at Waterloo, could afford an elaborately jointed, fruit-wood prosthesis – a handsome device that he displayed proudly to anybody who wanted to see the best that could be produced. So much did he value it that he insisted it be buried with him at Waterloo (his family later retrieved it for permanent exhibition in a family memorial).

The infamously celebrated procedure of 'blood-letting' (draining blood from cut veins) was a bizarre aberration of all logic and medical knowledge, even for the nineteenth century. It was somehow supposed to 'unload the blood vessels and relieve the circulation' of sick people, including the wounded. Neither theory had any possible credibility. The wonder is that it was continued for so long with absolutely no benefit and so much danger.

Enterprising doctors of the time gave their names to specially designed tools to bleed men. They created for them an aura of supreme knowledge despite the fact that the value of adequate circulation of the blood had been clearly explained by Harvey 150 years earlier. Used indiscriminately, blood-letting was frequently death dealing. Its absurd rationale was the exact opposite of what was recognised in the First World War, when substantial blood transfusion became a standard, high-priority treatment for the severely injured and shocked.

George Simmons of the 95th British Rifles was unlucky enough to be severely wounded by a musket ball at Waterloo. Although the ball was removed capably by his surgeon, the wound became deeply infected and he was soon moribund. During one four-day period, his surgeon slowly removed twelve pints of Simmons' blood, almost his total blood contents, relying on his body to manufacture more blood to replace the loss. He was so weak that he could no longer sit, stand or lift his head. If he had tried to stand, no doubt he would have fainted or died.

With no further surgical ideas springing to mind, a senior physician in private practice was called urgently into consultation. His astonishing suggestion? More letting of blood! This time, the incredible order was to be carried out by a generous application of leeches. Simmons was just alert enough to reject that suggestion and insist he be left to die; he wanted no more loss of blood.

For reasons best known to nature, within a week his wound began to discharge pus and his temperature fell. He recovered without further treatment and returned to light duties a month or so later, limited only by anaemia from loss of blood.

It is almost incredible that a lieutenant of infantry in a Napoleonic War could describe such a scene as this:

> I ... saw about 200 soldiers waiting to have their limbs amputated ... they had been wounded a week earlier ... their limbs were swollen enormously and the smell was dreadful ... some were sitting upright in the shade of trees ... many were wounded in the head as well as the limbs ... the poor fellows presented a dismal sight ... the streams of gore on their cheeks had been hardened by the sun and gave their faces a ... copper-coloured hue ... their eyes were sunk and fixed, resembling a group of bronze figures. They sat silent and statue like, waiting for their turn to be carried to the amputating tables.
>
> In an outer court were the surgeons. They were stripped to their shirts and bloody. To their right and left were arms flung here and there without distinction and the ground was dyed red ... a surgeon asked me to hold a man down while he removed his thigh ... the surgeon seemed insensible to the scene around him and was eating almonds out of his waistcoat pocket. The operation lasted half an hour but the man survived. To be able to administer ease and comfort to a victorious and heroic soldier had forged the sublimest pleasure that the mind of man is capable of enjoying.

It has taken many large and small wars for surgery to close the gap between those dark days and what modern combat hospitals can do, but the truth of the lieutenant's final comment endures.

A NEED FOR REGIMENTATION

Dr Michael E. DeBakey, a senior surgical consultant in the Second World War, frequently described how surgeons, suddenly confronted by many new and serious problems in war, also found themselves on foreign soil where men spoke with alien tongues. 'They needed to urgently learn to meet these conditions intellectually rather than emotionally,' he commented. Now they have become part of the military machine which relies on pragmatic, expedient, effective surgery matched precisely to the battle needs.

It was soon evident in the Second World War, and confirmed in later wars, that for armies to function well, casualties had to be treated quickly where they fell, then moved rapidly to more sophisticated treatment facilities. Once there, they could be given the necessary treatment to return them to possible battle capability. Additionally, troops had to be viewed as integral machines of war and treated for whatever else bothered them, separate from wounds, including whatever attributed to the preservation of morale.

None of these objectives could be realised without a high degree of uniformity in surgical management, even to the point of rigid standardisation of principles

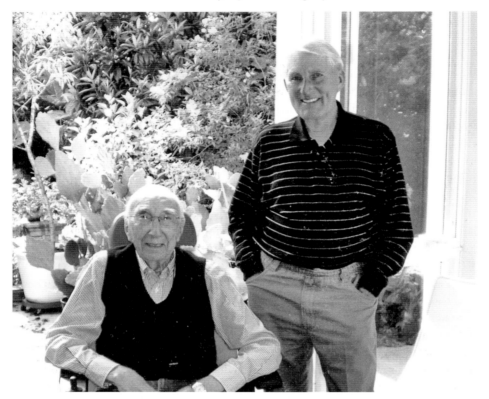

Dr Michael E. DeBakey, aged 99, an originator of 'MASH' forward surgical units, with the author in Houston, Texas, in September 2007. (*Dr J. Wright*)

and practices, and frank regimentation. Obviously, some 'free-wheeling' surgeons, freshly in combat areas from civilian life, found that irksome. It was found, for example, that after major injuries and surgery, troops did not travel well – despite this, they had to be entered as soon possible into an endless chain of evacuation out of the fighting zone. Every injured man and every surgeon had a rigidly apportioned position in the chain and was retained in that place unless there were a dire emergency that justified a short modification of the rules. Only then could surgeons assist the combative army. It followed that every staging post was equipped and staffed for a special function only and coordinated with every other post along the way.

A particular issue was the man in a combat area with a 'civilian-type' problem which affected his best function – such as a spinal disc or a knee ligament injury, a hernia, an abscess or appendicitis. Conventional ways of treating such conditions had to be streamlined to afford the best care most quickly with least loss of time from battle. By following pragmatic and uniform programs more than 500 years of hospital bed occupancy could be saved in one year alone.

None of these imposed surgical efficiency measures would have been completely effective were it not for the attention given to the very end of the chain – the expedited reception of wounded men into designated hospitals back home if they were not fit to continue in combat. In one period of the Second World War, between 1,000 and 3,000 such casualties were received every day and moved to an appropriate hospital within three days of arrival. Out of those momentous events, a great revision of the role, structure and integration of veterans' administration hospitals slowly evolved out of necessity. What also became evident very quickly was that injuries sustained in the later Pacific campaigns (though much less numerous than those from other major areas) did not arrive home in as good condition as those injured in Europe, the Mediterranean or North Africa. On the whole, this seemed due to a lack of senior surgeons and experienced anaesthetists in the Pacific, and a great difficulty in achieving uniformity in surgical procedures.

These difficulties were aggravated by the huge distances between island campaigns and, similarly, between them and the Australian and American hospitals that were receiving serious casualties. The surgical consultants formed the only consistent teaching facility that made effective 'regimentation' of surgical processes possible.

In Australia, five British medical officers were landed in Sydney with the 1788 First Fleet to pioneer trauma and other civilian treatment in the new colony. As the settlement expanded, various local garrisons and volunteer military medical groups were founded until, nearly 100 years later, Dr W. J. Bedford became the first staff surgeon supported by seventeen other surgeons. In 1885, a contingent of 700 Australian volunteers embarked for South Africa and the Sudan, including three doctors and five ambulance wagons powered by twenty-six horses.

In the 1890s, a well-organised New South Wales Medical Staff Corps was established, soon to be followed by other states providing contingents for the South African Wars of 1899. Four such groups were sent with establishments of medical officers, stretcher-bearers, ambulances, transports and horses able to sustain autonomous field hospitals. In 1900, the first ever Australian Victoria Cross was awarded to a medical officer, Captain Neville Howse.

ROYAL AUSTRALIAN ARMY MEDICAL CORPS (RAAMC)

By 1901, every state of the new Commonwealth of Australia was represented in Boer War contingents under Australian command, forming the Australian Army Medical Corps of 1902. At the 1914 outbreak of the First World War, it consisted of 187 medical officers and 1,678 other ranks who served with great distinction at Gallipoli and in Palestine, Syria and Europe.

A second Australian Imperial medical force was raised for the Second World War service in 1939 and served in the Mediterranean, North African, Middle

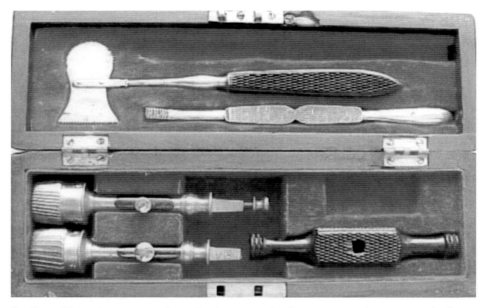

Skull trephining instruments from the American Civil War era, used to inspect the brain or drain the skull of fluids. Similar instruments were available thousands of years earlier. (*Dr M. Echols' collection*)

Eastern and South-West Pacific campaigns. Since the end of the Second World War, the RAAMC has seen further service in wars and peace-keeping missions involving Commonwealth forces in, among other places, Korea, Vietnam, Africa, the Middle East, Iraq, Afghanistan, Indonesia and Bougainville.

AUSTRALIAN MILITARY NURSES

In 1898, a small nursing service was established in Sydney, and some of the nurses later served with Australian troops in South Africa. Remarkably, little has been written of their gallant exploits then or, in fact, in many subsequent wars in which they have proved their immense value. Major-General Howse, VC, Director of Australian Medical Services after the First World War, is said to have regarded female nurses as nothing more than substitutes for trained, male orderlies – an opinion entirely contrary to the attitude of Field Marshal Montgomery in the Second World War.

Many nurses of both sexes and all countries have resented the poor recognition of their wartime contributions by official and unofficial war historians. Melanie Oppenheimer has called it the 'invisibility of women in war', pointing to the lack of their inclusion within the 'Anzac legend'. She observes that nurses' contributions were neglected during the commemoration of the ninetieth anniversary of Gallipoli in 2005, which concentrated on 'militarism, manhood and maleness'. She complains that Les Carlyon's history, *The Great War*, and the twelve-volume series, *Official History of Australia in the War of 1914–18*, excluded meaningful discussion of the roles of nurses. While, for reasons of safety, nurses were not allowed on the beaches of Gallipoli, they served with great distinction on hospital ships under heavy bombardment close by, and in hospitals in the Greek Islands, Malta and Egypt.

The Second World War saw more than 66,000 Australian women enlisted in auxiliary services alone, but they were rarely afforded equal recognition in ex-servicemen's groups. Oppenheimer perceives:

> We are all complicit in allowing women to be omitted from the dominant (male) war narrative; we have not raised our voices in protest nor have we questioned the writers, TV producers, journalists and politicians who continue to push this gender-based version of our history. On Remembrance Day perhaps we could focus on our service women and all women whose lives have been irreparably affected by war.

The First World War draft of Australian nurses departed in September 1914 for duties in Russia, Burma, the Middle East and Persian Gulf, Greece, Italy, France and England. By the end of the end of the war, many more than 2,000 of them had served overseas with Australian and British forces and 500 had served in Australia. Twenty-five died in service and nearly 400 were awarded military decorations.

Roslyn Bell and others have published extracts from the diaries and letters of some of these valiant women written during and after the First World War. Susanna de Vries has written extensively of the bravery and sacrifices of nurses who were with the AIF (Australian Imperial Force) in both world wars and mentions three female doctors who died during army service. Sister Elsie Gibson served on *Gascon*, anchored alongside another hospital ship, *Sicilia*, off Gallipoli on 25 April 1915, as it took on board more than 600 badly wounded men who arrived in an endless stream from the shore in any small boat that could accommodate them:

> When you see them brought in stretcher after stretcher in that endless procession and wonder if, when you see the next man's face, you will see one of your own friends, dear heaven, it's awful and every man or boy is somebody's boy.

Sister Alice Kitchen was wounded on board *Gascon* and her diaries refer to thirteen members of the Australian Army Nursing Service who died during the Gallipoli campaign.

Sister Ella Tucker was posted to *Gascon* for nine months as it ferried the wounded to various Mediterranean ports for intensive care after severe injuries, ultimately taking them to England:

> The wounded from the [Gallipoli] landing … poured into the ship's wards from barges and boats. The majority still had on their field dressings … two orderlies cut off the patients' clothes and I started immediately with dressings. There were 76 patients in my ward and I did not finish until 2 a.m. Every night there were two or three deaths, sometimes five or six … each night is a nightmare, the patients' faces … so pale with the flickering ship's lights.

Sister Lydia King was on the hospital ship *Sicilia*, off Gallipoli:

> I shall never forget the awful feeling of hopelessness in night duties … I had two wards downstairs, each over 100 patients, and then I had small wards upstairs – altogether about 250 patients to look after [with] one orderly and one Indian sweeper … the wounds were too awful. One loses sight of all the honour and the glory in the work we are doing.

Matron Grace Wilson and her staff of ninety-six nurses were posted to the island of Lemnos in August 1915 to receive the wounded from Gallipoli, despite having inadequate equipment and supplies:

> … found 150 patients lying on the ground … no equipment whatever … no water to drink or wash … a convoy arrived at night and used up all our private things, soap etc, tore up clothes for bandages … another convoy of about 400 [next day] just laid the men on the ground and gave them a drink. Very many badly shattered, nearly all stretcher cases … tents were erected over them as quickly as possible … all we can do is feed them and dress their wounds … a good many died … it is just too awful … one could never describe the scenes … could only wish [they had been] killed outright.

From a Casualty Clearing Station on the Western Front, a nurse described the scene before her:

> All the hospital lights were out … but the sky overhead was full of searchlights and fragments from the bursting anti-aircraft [shells] … I shall never forget the awful climb [out of a bomb crater] on hands and feet with greasy clay and blood … I kept calling for the orderly … but the poor boy had been blown to bits. When I tried to lift [another patient] with my arm under his leg, I found to my horror it was a loose leg with a boot and puttee on it … one of the orderly's legs which had been blown off … the next day they found his trunk about 20 yards away.

Sister Alys Ross sailed from Melbourne to Egypt on 21 November 1914 for service with one of the first Australian General Hospitals in Cairo. It received a constant stream of wounded from AIF desert camps and later, in Gaza, it received casualties from Gallipoli arriving in April 1915. She escorted many of the worst injured back to Australia on hospital ships before being sent to France with an Australian General Hospital to receive a torrent of devastation from the Western Front for the next fifteen months.

She recorded that German aircraft often ignored the red crosses of hospitals and bombed them heavily. In one such raid, she was stunned and shocked from bombs bursting around her, but was able to retreat to a tent. 'Though I shouted, nobody answered me or I could hear nothing for the roar of the planes and the artillery. I seemed to be the only living thing about.' She was awarded a Military Medal for her 'great coolness and devotion to duty'. During the third battle of Ypres, her Clearing Station was filled with wounded Australians, many of them doomed. 'The Last Post was being played nearly all day … so many dead.'

In November 1917, Alice returned to Rouen where she was senior nursing sister at an AGH. Later, she came across fifty-three badly wounded Germans who had been isolated and without water, food or care for three days. Thirteen died quickly:

I shall never forget the cries that greeted me … I got the doctor to come and fix them up … 40 patients in 45 minutes … no chloroform … amputations and all thirteen had died … onto the train an hour and a half after I found them.

CHAPTER 2

Surgery Comes of Age
with Anaesthesia

Despite their gadgets, and their ... augmented expertise, the anaesthetist [of the twentieth century] remained the genially despised 'rag-and-bottle man', bottle of chloroform in one tail pocket of his morning coat, square of lint to drip it upon in the other, the recipient of [only] ten per cent of the surgeon's fee ... the Jeeves of the operating theatre.

– Richard Gordon, *The Alarming History of Medicine*, St Martin's Press, 1993

Baghdad established a medical school in AD 765 and became the world's leading medical and pharmaceutical centre. The Arabic world already knew much about mood-altering drugs like opium, belladonna, cannabis and mandrake, whose derivatives are still used in pre-operative medication. But during the Crusades of AD 1000 and for close to another thousand years after, there was little advance in concepts of anaesthesia.[1] Men were gritting their teeth and writhing through their agony while surgeons and dentists were hastily attempting to make them better.

In AD 1288, an Arabian textbook made no mention of general anaesthesia, but referred to pain-killing medications and the need for powerful physical restraint during surgical operations. On both sides of the world there were references to large doses of alcohol and throttling of the carotid arteries in the neck to 'deaden the brain' – procedures which frequently led to temporary or even permanent coma. Some surgeons relied on the application of crushingly tight tourniquets to numb limbs to the point where the surgeon's knife was scarcely felt. Unfortunately, parts of the limbs often died just from the pressure of the tourniquets. Other surgeons bled patients until they lost consciousness – a most dangerous technique. Perhaps there was an advance in AD 1500 when Eastern authors described 'smothering' patients by sponges soaked in pungent

---

1. The first recorded general anaesthetics of comfortable, safe and predictable efficiency were given in about 1800 for civilians and soldiers, and extended slowly into wider military settings but with severe limitations in abdominal, brain and chest injuries. Sophisticated, curare relaxation 'arrived' slowly from 1815; opium analgesics in 1925; and the first truly effective hypnotic drug, pentothal, was not used extensively until 1941.

medications. They apparently produced sedation and pleasant hallucinations, but not a pain-free state. Opium and cannabis were repeatedly mentioned but, short of using deadly doses of those drugs, it seems that there was nothing much available to comfort during prolonged surgical procedures.

Relief would never have become possible without the means of profoundly and safely modifying consciousness with better drugs administered by better anaesthetists. Before the availability of general anaesthetics in England in about 1800, a famous London surgeon, Robert Liston, rivalled Larrey, the French surgical god, by amputating a leg from a wakeful patient in just a few minutes. On at least one occasion and in the presence of many observers, Liston was sketched removing the wrong leg in his haste to get on with the job. Just like a butcher of the time, he clamped his blood-soaked implements in his teeth in order to free his hands for the 'smash-and-grab' procedures which he performed to great applause. Like the Red Indians did on their tomahawks, he notched the handle of his knife to keep an accurate record of performances.

At the end of the eighteenth century, a chemist called Priestley discovered the pleasant, sedative effects of nitrous-oxide, commonly called 'laughing gas', because patients, as well as party-goers, felt very relaxed as they dozed-off under its influence. It was freely exploited as a recreational aid and as a general

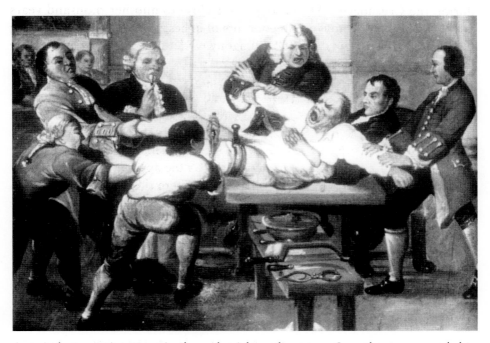

A typical amputation scene in the early eighteenth century. Several men are needed to restrain a patient without general anaesthesia. Note the tourniquet to control bleeding and surgical instruments. (*Unknown origin*)

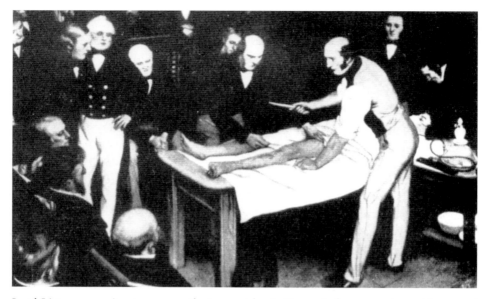

Lord Liston preparing to remove the 'wrong' leg in Europe's first operation with general anaesthetic, c. 1800. (*Richard Gordon*)

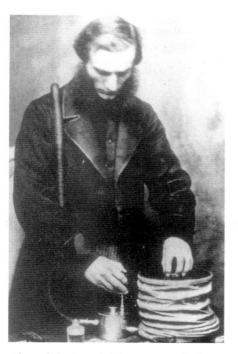

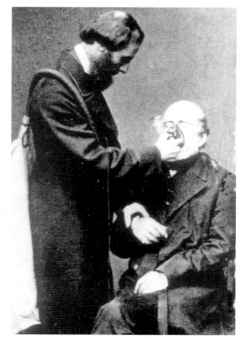

Above left: Joseph Clover, anaesthetist, prepares a chloroform gas delivery machine with 'banjo' ventilator device. (*Richard Gordon*)

Above right: Clover checks the patient's pulse as he administers the gas from a backpack through a mask. (*Richard Gordon*)

anaesthetic alongside liquid ether and chloroform. At that point, the whole nature of surgery in peace and in war was on the threshold of change. For the first time, surgeons could have comfortable working conditions with sleeping patients and relaxed muscles, despite whatever needed to be done to them.

In 1815, surgeons had also become aware of something called 'curare', a poisonous plant resin that was applied by South American Indians to their arrows and spears – it killed their enemies by paralysing their muscles. Its carefully controlled use, more than 100 years later, allowed much smaller and safer doses of 'sleep' drugs for anaesthesia because its relaxation of tight muscles allowed unrestricted surgical operations deep inside the body. For abdominal surgery (which carried the worst prognosis of all injured body regions) in particular, a new vista of possibilities was opened.

Regardless of new discoveries, ether remained cheaper and safer for the heart than chloroform but, unlike nitrous oxide and chloroform, it was dangerously inflammable and explosive. In a period when a naked flame was often used for illumination in surgical operations and bystanders chose to smoke their cigars and pipes as they observed proceedings, the safety benefits of using chloroform and nitrous oxide gas were obvious. (It is remarkable how many sketches of the time show well-dressed men observing surgical procedures as spectators – not assisting, just quietly chatting and smoking without apparent distress at what they were watching. It seems that operating was a very social affair.) At around that time, two American dentists were so impressed by the value of general anaesthesia in their work that they took out a patent for its use and received a notoriety they scarcely deserved.

The short-acting barbiturate, Pentothal, came much later but it remains the most popular sleep-inducing drug for every type of surgical procedure that requires unconsciousness. It is a remarkably useful anaesthetic because it needs no complicated apparatus except oxygen delivery and, when given by injection into a vein in proper dosage, it induces sleep in thirty seconds and lasts for about ten minutes – 'Just a prick in your wrist and you'll be asleep; when you wake up, you'll wonder if the job's been done.'

Although it had been discovered long before, Pentothal wasn't much used until the Japanese attack on Pearl Harbor in the Second World War. It was never meant to do more than provide rapid, pleasant sleep to begin formal anaesthesia. Then, other anaesthetic drugs, like ether and nitrous oxide, did the rest. It took time to learn that, in safe doses, Pentothal did not eliminate pain. (Lately, after many millions of successful administrations, the safety of nitrous oxide has also been questioned, but the evidence for doubts remains flimsy.)

It is astonishing that American anaesthetists introduced Pentothal widely before they were fully aware of how much to give and how frequently it should be given. The question of dosage was particularly significant when concerning severely injured patients whose circulation was disturbed by shock and whose bodies were in need of urgent and rapid anaesthesia. Pentothal's early reputation for being dangerous seems to have been more the result of how it was used, rather than testament to any innate danger. Its great advantage in war surgery is its rapid effect, sparing frightened, wounded soldiers the additional distress of inhaling unpleasant, sickly vapours in order to slowly reach oblivious sleep. For the same reasons it also has unique value in civilian surgery.

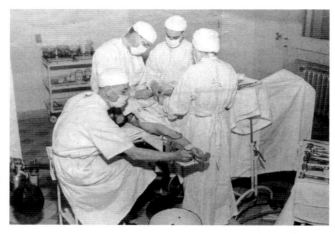

Surgeons and a nurse work with a typical Second World War general anaesthetic. Gas is administered by face mask and Pentothal is injected into the right arm. (*Surgical Consultants US Army, Second World War*)

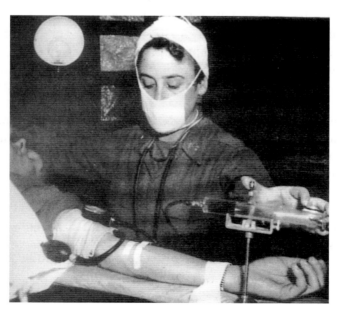

A nurse injecting Pentothal into a patient's left arm to begin anaesthesia, Second World War. (*US Army*)

CHAPTER 3

The Special Challenges of Military Medicine

I had neither medical orderlies nor stretchers. Not only was the hospital full of corpses, but so were the streets and a number of the houses ... on my own I took away 128 of them which were serving as pillows to the sick, and were already several days old.

– Russian surgeon, The Grande Armée, 1812

It is not up to the surgeon to determine whether a wound is self-inflicted. That role belongs to a judge. A doctor must be his patient's friend. He must look after both the guilty and the innocent and concentrate his efforts solely on the injury. The rest is not his business.

– Baron Dominique-Jean Larrey, 1807, according to Professor M. Feinsod

The standardisation of medical care is made difficult by the variable demands and locations of war, especially with the advent and multiplication of new and more complicated weapons. Doctors needed to adapt to the new means of killing and maiming – both military and civilian – as quickly as possible. Inevitably, individual and collective military consciences have been challenged throughout history and tormenting issues remain for all medical carers to confront.

Military medicine was once regarded as a special interest for some surgeons and physicians – something to do on weekends and vacations, and in wartime. Today, it is a super speciality in its own right. Unlike civilian hospitals, many military units are semi-permanent – either completely or partly mobile. All concentrate on the treatment of mass casualties by the principles of triage. Civilian hospitals work in a formal triage mode only in the event of major civilian or terrorist disasters.

Army hospitals were first developed in Greece as long ago as 500 BC. The idea was taken up by the Romans who built them specifically for their veterans. In the seventeenth century, Renaissance armies appointed untrained and unwilling surgeons to service poorly equipped field units where the doctors exhibited poor medical care and standards of hygiene. In those unpopular places, diseases spread uncontrollably, but at least they were the beginnings of better things for injured fighting men and their medical helpers.

By the second half of the nineteenth century, anti-tetanus serum was widely available and hospital and medical care, anaesthesia and recovery rates had improved to the point where clean surgical procedures under general anaesthesia were the rule. At the instigation of Florence Nightingale, the British reformed the training of nurses and hospital orderlies and established sanitary commissions. The fighting world soon followed Germany in developing a logical chain of evacuation of the wounded from regimental aid posts through dressing stations to casualty clearing stations, then on to field hospitals and, finally, general hospitals far behind the combat lines. At last, progress was developing in such a way as to encourage doctors to take up a military life that provided infrequent combat practice, but also high authority in the event of war.

The development of trench warfare secured the infantryman as the most vital and vulnerable element of combat, but the First World War demonstrated a lack of adequate medical expertise in the field and, even more, a pressing need for a rapid evacuation formula. The foot soldier witnessed these deficiencies all too clearly, particularly in the trenches. He was a beast of burden, laden with rifle, ammunition and pack, endangered in the trenches by enemy artillery and, all too often, the 'friendly fire' of his own army's guns. He marched long distances through all terrains and climates, often wondering why he was there, where he was going and what would happen to him if injured. A satisfactory answer to his last and most pressing question had to await the advent of rapid first aid and helicopter transportation decades later.

In 1915, a new and appalling means of warfare emerged. Allied soldiers were poisoned with German chlorine, phosphorus and mustard gas for the first time. When the wind was favourable to the aggressor, a cloud of toxic fumes was released to waft across enemy lines. Without effective masks, the only refuge with partial safety was to lie flat on the ground, below the gas cloud, and hope it did little harm. With their first gas attack, Germany left 5,000 Allied soldiers dead and dying, and 10,000 others disabled for life.

Rob Ruggenberg, Dutch journalist and First World War enthusiast, reports that thousands of live, rusting gas cylinders and shells from the First World War are still piled up in the Belgian countryside. Many more canisters are buried around beaches and rivers where they slowly corrode and release their deadly contents into the sea. Although they were not directly involved in their wartime use, five distinguished German medical scientists who helped develop these gases were rewarded with Nobel Prizes.

By the time of the Normandy invasion in 1944, military medicine had transformed itself greatly. For each British division of 16,000 men, there were 25,000 non-combatants in support, including more than 1,000 medical personnel. In Vietnam sixteen years later, it was estimated that for every soldier,

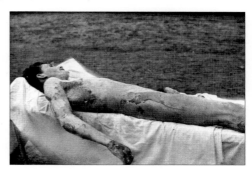

The untreatable effects of mustard gas
burns, First World War. (*R. Ruggenberg*)

sailor or airman in active combat, there were ten individuals backing him up
– the most important being the rapid salvage teams and specialists in major
hospitals. Even so, wounds to the head, chest and particularly the abdomen
still carry by far the highest mortality rate of all areas of injury, despite vast
improvements in specialist practice over the last century.

As a continuing worldwide threat, there are more than 500 million 'small'
arms in constant international circulation today, causing at least one death
somewhere in the world every forty seconds of every year. Inevitably, medical
teams in combat zones are involved in treating the slaughtered victims of an
arms trade that carries little or no personal, corporate, commercial or national
risk to the merchants. It is very steady work with inherent taxation advantages,
operated from afar by unscrupulous salesmen. Health teams find it impossible
to provide and maintain effective medical services in all the countries in which
they are deployed. The manufacturers profit from both the death and the
endless misery they knowingly produce.

It is often overlooked that through the centuries doctors, nurses and their
colleagues have treated wounded enemy troops as well as their own. Even
today, they treat terrorists and innocent civilians who have medical conditions
unrelated to armed conflict. With the improvements in battlefield evacuation,
surgical teams working behind the front line often have to perform a torrent
of life-saving surgical amputations for troops who might once have died from
their injuries. In confronting these ugly tasks, medical teams perform their
duties for long hours in conditions of maximum stress. They are often isolated,
working with unfamiliar colleagues in places and countries they would never
have chosen to visit. Most medical personnel derive a great sense of purpose
in what they do, whether or not they get the help and respect they deserve.
Unbelievably, the vast majority operating in warzones work unarmed, with
little or no personal protection and almost no public recognition.

Medical morale is probably at its lowest in regions affected by civil
war, displacement and famine. In the Darfur region of Sudan, hundreds
of thousands of civilians will die or have to flee unless large UN military
teams can make it safe for doctors and other volunteers to work for long,

unbroken periods. Whatever support there is, it is inadequate, belated or remote.

It is a feature of modern life that public morale can only be maintained by sustained and unstinting press coverage. On the other hand, medical staff see that the media's insatiable hunger to infiltrate hospitals and operating rooms to observe spectacular drama is highly selective. Just now, Africa is not a primary interest. In collecting material for worldly consumption, media contact is largely confined to the more insulated 'green zones' of combat, causing some ostensibly independent information to be non-sequential, second-hand or medically and factually inaccurate. That doesn't stop heavily negative stories getting wide exposure and altering domestic opinion. As a result, medical workers often find that coverage of that type becomes unhelpful to them and all those who believe in what they are doing, as well as to those who rely on their help.

In discussing the special circumstances of combat surgery and the complex compromises in care, Greg Zoroya has identified an unusual and, probably, new dilemma confronting surgeons and other health workers. It arises when high degrees of technical success create an ethical ambivalence – a striving to preserve lives which are so damaged that some might doubt that they are worth saving. Very obviously, a neurosurgeon may be confronted with profound questions in the case of severe, irrecoverable brain damage. One justification for preservation at any cost is to allow families to share the ultimate responsibility for decision-making. Increasingly, these have become matters for next of kin to contemplate when severely injured troops are repatriated to die at home.

All surgeons soon discover that the reality of the battlefield is different from anything they have ever experienced before – nastier, more depressing and needing a higher level of pragmatism, especially when medical services are made available to injured prisoners. A surgeon may have to confront his own troops' arguments against the notion of saving the lives of enemy soldiers – especially failed suicide terrorists or 'civilians' who may have recently killed a surgeon's friends. Most find discrimination unethical and intuitively unacceptable but nevertheless very difficult to avoid.

Not surprisingly, many surgeons and their teams are initially apprehensive about their ability to handle the extraordinary pressures of combat surgery. In Iraq, one took to wearing a combat helmet in the operating room and another carried a small pistol constantly. Others ran endless marathons in the desert at night or worked out in gymnasiums to keep their minds off the next day's horrors. An older surgeon wore combat goggles containing a prescription for his astigmatism. He commented during a very challenging operation that, '[We all have to deal with] tremendous amounts of bleeding, tremendous amounts of injury ... all I can do is the best I can do ... I couldn't sleep if I didn't.'

Richard Hyer of *Medscape Medical News* recently reported the observations of Dr Paul Cordts who served in Iraq, where most battle wounds are now

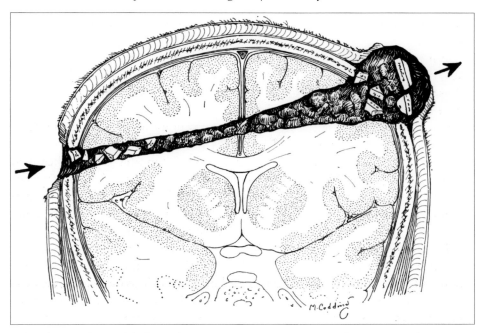

A 'through-the-head' injury with massive brain damage and skull fragmentation. The question is: should surgeons attempt anything? (*Dr M. Crumplin*)

due to improvised explosive devices (IEDs). So rapidly are wounded men evacuated to surgical care that the rates of death during or soon after surgery have actually increased in Balad Hospital. Within an hour of injury, men are now dying of hopelessly untreatable wounds inside operating rooms, instead of in the field. Cordts praises the latest body-armour which provides better protection for the chest and abdomen, with supplementary plates being developed for the neck, shoulders and groins.

There has been a disquieting recent finding of a relatively high frequency of deep vein thrombosis (DVT) in young men, not only in those with major lower limb injuries. These days, all soldiers carry a first-aid kit containing a tourniquet, pressure dressings and special new bandages containing shell-fish products, which hasten control of bleeding from large surface wounds. While these materials are life saving, there is some concern that their clot-promoting properties might be a factor in the increasing frequency of DVT.

The Supreme Allied Commander in the Second World War, General Dwight Eisenhower, later the thirty-fourth US President, said in 1953 what every medical worker believes: 'Every gun that is made, every warship launched, every rocket fired, signifies a theft from those who hunger and are not fed, those who are cold and are not clothed.' Fifty years later, UN Secretary Kofi Annan was even more specific: 'The death toll from small arms dwarfs that of all other weapons systems – and in most years greatly exceeds the toll of the

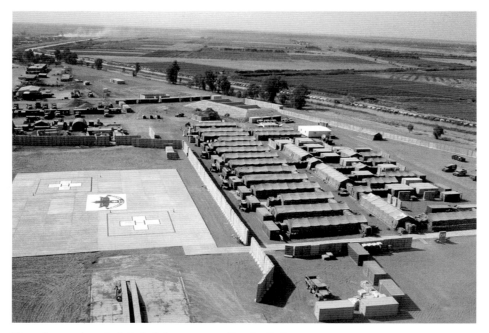

Tented army hospital, Balad, Iraq, 2008. (*Dr G. K. Bruce*)

atom-bombs that devastated Hiroshima and Nagasaki. In terms of the carnage they cause, small arms, indeed, could well be described as the "weapons of mass destruction".'

Much war surgery is depressing, tedious and unglamorous. There is a sameness in what the public sees and hears of the situations in Iraq and Afghanistan, where most carnage is related to ethnic conflict and a lack of security against radical insurgents. Only the numbers and details of the tragedies change. Media coverage has become repetitive while there is little mention of much worse devastation elsewhere in the world – especially in Africa.

The medical problems of Iraq remain extreme: civilian hospitals buy protection from armed gangs by employing their own armed gangs; surgeons travel to work in inconspicuous, armour-plated vehicles to avoid detection; while some have been murdered in the streets or in their homes and hospitals. The question is why and for how long doctors can continue?

THE PROMISE OF MULTI-SKILLING

Most of the American public does not know that civilian trauma is the leading cause of death for those aged one to 34. Most are confident of receiving the best medical care in the event of serious injury. But only eight states have fully developed trauma systems. Ninety percent of Americans believe that their hospitals should all have a coordinated trauma response system. This has not been made a national priority.

– Champion *et al.*, 2006

Guerrillas and terrorists are the new faces of warfare. Every year, firearms used in anger kill 500,000 people, half of them in war and half in civilian life. The salvage surgery of combat has spawned another new race of young, predominantly male survivors who are substantially maimed – missing limbs, disfigured, impotent, blind, disturbed and unstable, needing some degree of life-long special care.

This has flowed predictably from the nature of new wars and weapons and, ironically, from the excellence of early medical care. Salvage of even grossly impaired life has become an aim of military healthcare and conventional triage has had to radically change its rules. Today, there is a new sort of survivor, who carries an awful disability home to a confused and frightened family.

To advance those issues, specialised faculties of 'trauma' are being developed in affluent countries. Their target is the multi-skilling of surgeons, nurses and other medical personnel to best manage any sort of catastrophe, civilian or military. An example arose in 1944 when the Birmingham Accident Hospital in England opened its doors and set out to express an ideal – to treat only trauma victims. The impetus for the hospital, which rapidly became an international benchmark, lay in a perceived inadequacy of treatment of the seriously injured throughout the British Isles, particularly civilian and military victims of the Second World War.

Birmingham had three trauma teams, each consisting of two consultant surgeons, a consultant anaesthetist, nurses, physiotherapists and other support services involved in trauma care. They also had a dedicated burns team with three specialist surgeons. The surgical teams were responsible for patients throughout their entire treatment – hospital, recovery and rehabilitation. The last was an integral part of the program. Inevitably, all staff members rapidly became familiar with what their colleagues were doing and why. Other countries quickly followed Birmingham's lead. With the advent of the National Health Service in Britain in 1948, the government was seeking economies wherever it could find them. The result was that the Birmingham unit began to be decommissioned almost as soon as it began, until it ceased to exist in 1993. The British government had decided that the same work could be done adequately in many general hospitals. In its absence, the number of British and Commonwealth surgeons able to manage 'all-weather, any-time, go-anywhere' surgery dwindled.

Fortunately for others, the departed icon of trauma surgery had left its mark. In the US, designated trauma centres promoted by the American College of Surgeons had been established in 1971, and it has been left to American and continental surgeons to widely demonstrate the value of multi-skilling in recent and current wars.

So intent have the Americans been on giving best care to the 80 per cent of casualties in Iraq and Afghanistan who are not able to return to military duties, that they have recently established four 'poly trauma' centres strategically placed throughout the country. They are staffed by doctors whose jobs include the identification and care of occult brain dysfunction, which may show itself by defects of speech, movements, hearing, vision, memory, reasoning and other less obvious markers of brain damage, most of which has been blamed on blast trauma from IEDs.

Another retrograde step in valuable established principles has affected military hospitals in Britain. From the days of Florence Nightingale, service men and women have been treated in designated centres. Lately, those centres have also been closed down in a further process of rationalisation of resources. With those economies, service personnel are increasingly apprehensive about the quality of their care and their priority for special attention when they are returned to civilian life or convalescence. Veterans justifiably wonder why they can no longer have the same standard of care that they experienced in military hospitals.

AUSTRALIAN REGIMENTAL MEDICAL OFFICERS

Regimental Medical Officers (RMOs) accompany fighting units and attend to the immediate needs of troops, whether that be daily medical maintenance or combat wounds in the front line. They are the carers responsible for life-and-death decisions from the earliest moments of conflicts. Without them, nothing could be accomplished quickly and with perspective.

In 1940, only eighteen months after his graduation, one Australian doctor, who wishes to be anonymous, enlisted in the AIF with no more military experience than a few years of spare-time service in the Sydney University Regiment. Within a few months and with no formal course of training or surgical knowledge, he was sent to Darwin as an RMO to an infantry battalion of 400 men. With no nurses, medical colleagues or accessible superior military officers, he taught a small group of stretcher-bearers the elements of first aid, how to mix morphine in a spoon and how to apply a Thomas splint. Just as he wondered what on earth was happening to him, a waterside workers' strike meant the battalion was sent to unload ships waiting in Darwin Harbour. When that was over, his further medical activity consisted of dispensing condoms, 'short-arm parades' (inspecting penises for venereal disease), painting sore throats with a soothing concoction that lasted about fifteen minutes, putting useless powders and creams on rashes, treating sunburn and supervising sick parades for soldiers who weren't really sick at all.

Late in 1940, the order suddenly came for the RMO to return to Sydney by flying boat post-haste and prepare to leave for the Middle East on the *Queen Mary*. He recalled that there were five other passenger liners also fitted out for transporting Australian troops. On board, he met other medical officers whose experience up to that point had been as frustrating as his. When they arrived at Ceylon, smaller ships took them on to Palestine where they were assembled near Gaza for overland trucking to Libya. His only medical activities during those movements consisted of the same tedious, 'civilian-type' medical care for troops, whose trivial complaints were in no way military in nature. That reinforced his sense of futility about what he might meaningfully contribute to the war effort.

The Australian 6th Division and the British had left North Africa to defend Greece, where they sustained enormous losses. The RMO's group was to replace them in North Africa, mopping up Italian stragglers and moving in a wide sweep towards Tobruk through Libya's western desert. There were few other doctors and no surgeons available to his battalion, which travelled vast distances across uncharted desert by night in crowded trucks and with little idea of what would next happen to them. By April 1941, they knew that Rommel's troops were also aiming for Tobruk and his battalion watched the approaching Germans from the Australian-held escarpment. The RMO, now a captain, occasionally saw Australians with bomb injuries to their limbs, but they were rapidly transferred east to Tobruk where there were substantial surgical resources.

His own medical capabilities had not been enhanced in any way since he left Sydney and his menial medical duties continued without supervision or promise of change. To gain immunity from physical harm in the event of being captured, he never carried a weapon despite being increasingly aware of intensive fighting nearby. None of it involved him because he was told to stay far behind the combat lines; back there, he was never fired at or bombed and despite having a car and a driver, he found his isolated situation increasingly frustrating. His few medical talents were ignored.

As his battalion finally entered Tobruk, they learned that many Australians had been captured by the Germans. The Australian contingent was disorganised and retreating from the German advance, moving into the relative shelter of Tobruk. On arrival and with no clear direction from superior officers, the RMO was left to his own meagre resources – no antibiotics, little blood and no nurses working in his area. By attaching himself to a Field Ambulance and Casualty Clearing Station, he observed men with bomb injuries and, for the first time, began to believe that he might yet be of some use to the army, if only as an observer and dressings-changer.

A major assault on the city was expected on Easter Sunday, 1941, but when it came, the initial German attack was repulsed by the Australian 9th Division and a few British units. Tobruk was tightly besieged and, for many months, it was defended by Australian infantry.

After three months of hard conditions – where flies were a constant problem – the RMO experienced severe, unremitting dysentery which left him dehydrated, undernourished and needing hospital care. He was moved to a well-equipped hospital on the Mediterranean Coast, west of Tobruk township, and was immediately declared unfit for any further service. He was told to get aboard an Australian destroyer in Tobruk Harbour for evacuation to Alexandria. From there he was sent home, arriving back in Sydney in September 1941, a few months before the Japanese entered the war.

Discharged 'medically unfit' for further active service, but without any firm diagnosis apart from exhaustion and slowly recovering dysentery, the RMO left the army to take up a training post in Brisbane. When large numbers of wounded men from New Guinea and other South-West Pacific campaigns began to arrive in Australia, he rejoined the army and served as a physician in several 1,000-bed military hospitals in Queensland and New South Wales until 1945. He then resumed civilian life as a specialist and worked in distinguished centres overseas until his retirement twenty years ago.

So, what is his place in the vast and complex mosaic of military service? Today, at the age of ninety-two, he grieves that his time and talents were squandered because he was never trained, supported, advised or valued. It seems extraordinary that he was accepted into the army when, just out of medical school, he had so little to offer in the way of experience. Yet, he ended up in Tobruk under siege and looks back with regret. They were lost and traumatic years for a young doctor of untapped talents, an 'exercise in failure of planning' and none of it his fault.

The experiences of another RMO, Dr Philip Thomas – also without significant surgical expertise – began in Western Australia in November 1939. Ultimately, he spent five years in the Mediterranean, North Africa and the Middle East. Much of his work was the same sort of hum-drum activity described above. At first, he saw little fighting and witnessed much confusion in command directions. What he considered to be, for him, a 'phoney war' in the Middle East continued until December 1940, when he was assigned to 'real' doctoring and treating casualties in the Western Desert and the later disastrous campaigns in Greece and Crete.

Shortly after the Pearl Harbor attack on 7 December 1941, he was returned to Western Australia before being posted to New Guinea in 1943. There he experienced many cases of malaria and typhus, but had few drugs to treat them. After six months, he was promoted to the rank of Lieutenant-Colonel and returned to Australia in charge of a convalescent hospital in Western Australia. He was discharged unfit with an eye disease in late 1944.

His contributions were great, attending to many troops, often with relatively minor but important 'fitness' disorders, most of them unrelated to combat. His observations suggested that much of his work was frustrating, uninteresting and performed in many locations, giving him only a limited sense of responsibility and significance. Nevertheless, somebody had to deliver the sort of care that he had given through five years of service.

Dr H. D. 'Blue' Steward spent his Second World War service as the RMO of 2/16th Battalion in Syria, the Middle East and on the Kokoda Trail – the 'coldest, wettest jungle in the world'. He acknowledged the superb assistance of the Papuan natives, who carried wounded men for as long as ten days. The undernourished Australian foot soldiers carried their 20 kilograms of personal equipment up and down the treacherous paths, often at a cold altitude where, though free of mosquitoes and malaria risk, their energy was sapped. Steward had found malaria a serious problem in Port Moresby, where there was a mortality rate of 25 per cent and few anti-malarial drugs were available. No penicillin was provided until 1944. His staff carried no guns or ammunition, but had heavier loads of medical equipment, including serum and plasma.

When the Japanese finally retreated to the north coast of Papua in November 1942, some rest and recuperation was possible for the Australians who were exhausted from lack of sleep, 'trench foot', malaria and dysentery. Steward attributed much of their 'war neurosis' to a combination of boredom, fear, isolation, loneliness, the 'nostalgia' described by the Swiss in the First World War, and strained relationships between troops and their leaders. He was convinced that the maintenance of morale was essential to avoid dementia and death among the most distressed.

In early 1943, Steward became severely ill from dysentery and returned to Australia. His descriptions of conditions on the Kokoda Trail reveal the extraordinary demands on both doctors and troops and his own great humanity and frustration. He tells of seeing:

... a 23 year old former golf professional [with] a ghastly, gaping wound of the throat and, although my eyes could see only darkness and death, he saw light and hope. They were asking me something with all the mute urgency that eyes can convey ... every facet of the inner feelings – love, joy, hope, fear, guilt, pity, hatred ... emotion clouds calm clinical judgement but the hardest thing is to not flinch from the gaze of the man you know is going to die.

Evacuation by helicopter [as later in Vietnam] or ... a surgical team nearby might have given him a fighting chance. But I could do so little and here we were, cut off without certainty of getting out at all ... but there was Private Roy Turner, an indomitable stretcher bearer... who hoisted that man across his shoulders and carried him out ... to no avail.

The scene on board the ship returning Stewart to Moresby on New Year's Eve 1942 was different but no less graphic as he saw it:

... none of the hearty deck games that would have been played if we had been outward bound to battle ... the fever cases ... still struggled with their sweats and rigors ... miserable in the confinement of the ship so we ... brought them up on deck, eyes bleared by fever-haunted sleep catching the first grey of dawn at sea ... the facts, sounds, smells and sights both beautiful and horrible, the words, voices, the feel of ooze underfoot and the wetness gluing the clothes to your skin ... all these things were instantly in my mind when ... we made our Australian landfall ... the ship's funnel [filling] the sky with sparks.

CHAPTER 4

Gunpowder and its Progeny

I have prepared one of my own time capsules ... and have placed some rather large samples of dynamite, gunpowder and nitro-glycerine [in it]. My time capsule is set to go off in the year 3000. It will show them what we are really like.

– Alfred Hitchcock, US film director 1899–1980

Whether or not the Chinese or the Arabs or Friar Berthold Swartz (who probably never existed) originated its application to guns, there is no doubt that gunpowder did lead to artillery and bombs, which led to modern surgery. No single thing has more influenced the history and affairs of nations and of surgery over the last 600 years than the gun. It allowed Europeans to defeat the Africans and white Americans to defeat the Red Indians.

In its earliest days, what became known as 'gunpowder' was first used as a medication for wounds, infections and snakebites, but there is no evidence that it was useful for any of those problems. Ambroise Paré, a French surgeon of the sixteenth century, was confident that adding it and boiling oil to an early recipe of eggs, rosewater, turpentine, puppy fat, worms and the oil of lilies, would cleanse wounds of infection. The concoction proved useless.

How somebody might have discovered that the addition of potassium nitrate (saltpetre) to a mixture of charcoal and sulphur created a mix which exploded when compressed or ignited, is an insoluble riddle. How somebody then discovered that gunpowder exploding within a tube could expel a missile at killing speed is not quite so baffling. And so a brand-new weapon called a gun became the instrument of man's destructive impulses.

By the end of the fifteenth century, gunshot wounds had become the largest military blight on mankind. To make matters worse, in 1850 nitro-cellulose was added to gunpowder to make its explosion even more violent. Soon after, dynamite and gelignite for war came onto the market freely. Ten years later, Alfred Nobel, the originator of the Nobel Prizes, was busily experimenting with a nitro-glycerine compound while isolated on a raft moored, for safety's sake, in the middle of the River Elbe in Germany. Through his experiments, he dramatically advanced the tools of killing.

Some may think it a pity that he didn't destroy himself and his invention, but instead he demonstrated that TNT (tri-nitro-toluene) was the most powerful explosive of that time. Exploiting the inventiveness of the jolly British general, Henry Shrapnel, Nobel's destructive genius had enabled cannon balls, incendiaries, grape-shot, chain-shot and exploding shells to wreak unheard-of damage to wide areas around the impact site. Perhaps his donation of peace prizes was meant to soothe his shame of the monster he had fathered.

Between the world wars, armouries were further enhanced by rapid-firing artillery which could accurately send shells containing all sorts of death-dealing substances for 30 miles. Many of their targets never knew where the missiles had originated or when they were coming. That was exceptionally destructive for the nerves of fearful, isolated troops, and for their surgeons as they anxiously awaited vast new waves of pulverised soldiers.

More recently, the munitions industry has created even more hideous monsters in cluster bombs and inflammable vapour such as were used in Vietnam, Afghanistan and Chechnya. The heat, blast and solid missiles can

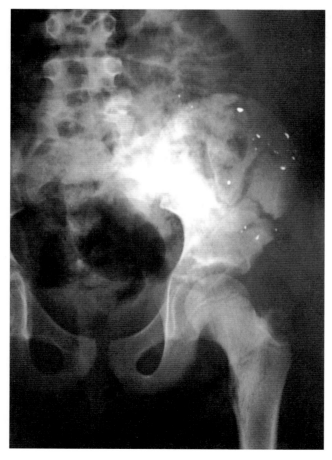

Shattered right pelvic bone with scattered metallic fragments. (US Army)

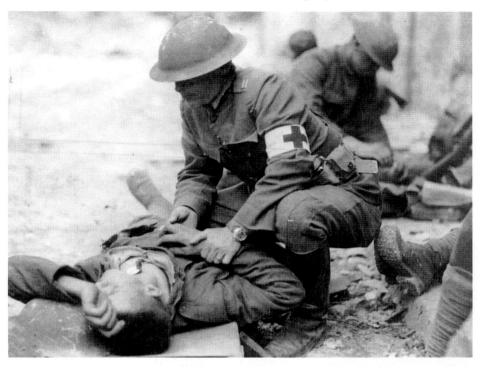

Men gassed by uncontrollable wind delivery, First World War. Lung damage prevented their return to battle and frequently caused lifelong disability. (*R. Ruggenberg*)

destroy everything in range, regardless of protective shields, adding the resulting injuries to the challenges of modern surgical techniques.

All weapons may carry or produce toxic materials that kill if inhaled or come into contact with skin. Their ultimate medical effects are unpredictable and uncontrollable, but few have much surgical relevance as almost all are totally beyond curing. They can destroy the continuity and integrity of all body structures. Explosives such as the 12-kiloton Hiroshima and Nagasaki atomic bombs had blast effects equivalent to many tons of TNT. Their enormous blast waves introduced a new dimension – the potential for planetary destruction.

MODERN TIMES

Because they are flexible, liquid or elastic, 'plastic' explosives such as Semtex (once used extensively by the Provisional IRA) and C-4 are terrorists' favourites. They are the explosive components of the easily portable weapons which have created devastating challenges for surgical teams everywhere. Terrorists used Semtex in the destruction of a military complex in Saudi Arabia in 1996, and in an attack on the American ship USS *Cole* in 2000. C-4 has been used in suicidal bombings in Israel and is favoured by al-Qaeda. It comes in malleable sticks and can be moulded into any shape. It was ideal, therefore, for the British bomber who had 10 ounces of it in each shoe when he boarded a flight in Paris in 2001, intent on suicidal destruction. Further afield, Indonesian police found traces of C-4 at the Bali bomb scene in 2002.

These explosives are manufactured not only in the United States but also in the Balkans, from where they have been purchased by Islamic militants in recent years. Alongside those more sophisticated 'personal' explosives, many commercially available nitrate-containing compounds allow terrorists to domestically fabricate bombs of huge power, such as those being used in IEDs in Iraq and Afghanistan. It is often claimed that 'smart' weapons are precision instruments, which carry fewer risks for civilians. While they may be smart by making war safer for the military, many believe that they are not smart enough to avoid devastating damage to civilian establishments that may be mistaken for military installations and ordnance. The amount of 'collateral damage' resulting from such 'discriminating' weapons deployed from remote sites depends on the quality of intelligence, communications and guidance that goes into their use. The intelligence available to those who fire the weapons

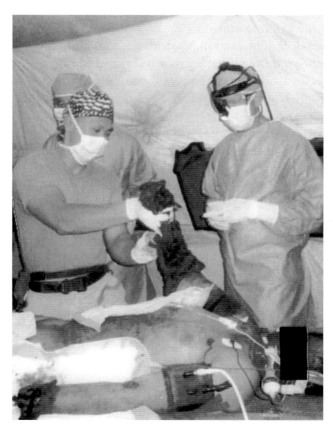

Destruction of both upper limbs by an Improvised Explosive Device (IED). (*Dr G. Peoples*)

is often faulty or out-of-date – hence, their damage may be surprisingly widespread.

As always, survival from collateral damage is related directly to the accuracy of aim and the radius of destruction of these weapons. Similar to the long-range artillery and scatter bombing of the First World War, remotely-originating, anonymous weapons raise the question of whose legal and moral responsibility it is for injuries resulting from them. For the surgeon, of course, the physical harm inflicted on casualties is no less, and perhaps worse because of the disintegrative effects of modern rockets directed at small targets.

A forensic scientist told *The London Times* how he felt about domestic bomb makers:

> You keep hearing that terrorists can easily make a bomb from using instructions on the internet. You can, but not of the design and sophistication of these devices [found in London]. These were well put together ... the bomb maker had highly developed skill.

When traces of military plastic explosives were found in the debris of wrecked underground carriages and a bus in London in 2005, it was concluded that one individual had probably assembled all four devices. Furthermore, the triggering devices used in the London suicide attacks were almost identical to those found in the rucksack bombs used in Madrid in 2004, although the latter contained industrial dynamite stolen from a quarry in Spain rather than plastic explosives. Investigators discovered that the London bombs were detonated by synchronised alarms from mobile telephones, as they were in Madrid, or by wristwatch alarms.

How the explosives were procured remains a mystery, but all agreed with McGrory and Evans that it was urgent to find the mastermind behind these explosives. When Scotland Yard investigated military bases and building sites around Europe, it came up with the disturbing conclusion that most modern military explosives are hard to detect by X-rays, easy to hide, stable until triggered and, if contained in a drum, may evade explosive-sniffing dogs and other detection devices.

Dr Andrew Dearden later described his sickening experience as he left a surgical meeting at the British Medical Association building during the London bombings in July 2005:

> ... I heard a loud 'whomping' ... I thought it may have been a crash but the sound was very loud – a big sound that resonated ... I saw the bus site about 20 metres away ... scattered glass and metal fragments ... I could see pieces of materials and people's possessions strewn around. I saw a woman's purse. Then I ran past a dismembered limb on the ground and noticed other parts of human bodies. Three of my most vivid images of the day were the bus, the

purse and the limb ... doctors were tending people on the ground, a severe leg injury difficult to bandage because it was so severe, putting drips into the arms of the dying, giving oxygen ... so busy there was no time to talk, hours passed in minutes ... we were able to keep people alive long enough to make repairs possible ... I felt as if I was in a bubble ... some of the people I had seen that morning would never be able to walk again ... twelve hours later I was drained of all my strength ... you do the doctoring and deal with the emotion and pain of it later.

Nurse Angie Scarisbricke was also caught up in one of the new civilian battle zones that have replaced conventional war sites. On the same day, she heard and saw the results of an explosion on a bus in Tavistock Square. She later saw some of the wounded lined up for urgent surgery by hastily assembled surgeons who worked non-stop and simultaneously until all the injured had been treated as well as possible. These weren't the sorts of procedures they were used to:

... a big bang ... workmen running down the street ... gruesome scenes of shocked people covered in ash ... people deafened by blasted eardrums, others unable to see ... a man with a severed leg, a woman with a severed foot ... [I'm] ... attending to a cardiac arrest.

The Reverend Brian Lee is neither a military padre nor a chaplain. He heard the bomb detonated in the tube between Aldgate and Liverpool Street stations as he was walking to his church. He tried to comfort some of the walking wounded in the vicinity, just as his battle colleagues have been doing for centuries:

You just sit with someone and hold their hands and be still and be with them. There's no need to say anything; just being there for them is the main thing ... then the mobile phone lines went down ... the church became a command centre and was opened as a rest centre for rescue workers, open 24 hours ... it wouldn't be right to say that the bombing made me question my belief in God. The spirit that I kept seeing in those rescue workers has encouraged me and reaffirmed my faith ... [in the evening] the emergency services went down to the tracks to remove the bodies of the dead passengers ... they asked me to accompany them, which I did ... I asked God to watch over [the dead] and said the words of The Lord's Prayer over and over.

CHAPTER 5

Body-Armour

Modern body-armour may combine a ballistic vest, a combat helmet, ballistic shoulder and side armor [and] face and spine protection. Soft vests are worn by police, private citizens, security and body-guards. Hard plate reinforced vests are worn by combat soldiers, police and hostage rescue teams.

– Wikipedia

Ancient Egyptian surgeons were sufficiently concerned with the avoidance of head injuries that they recommended the use of military helmets. Later combatants aimed to protect the whole body by flexible armour made of chain or plate-mail, augmented by a portable, protective shield. Various modifications followed, always seeking greater lightness and flexibility but, eventually, gunpowder overcame light armour to become the overpoweringly successful villain of war. Its effects usually defeat even carefully designed body-armour systems.

In the First World War, the steel helmet was the basic protection in all armies; nothing was added until the Second World War when some form of whole-body protection became a high priority, at least for the US Army. Flak-jackets became available only towards the end of the Second World War, but they came too late for use in significant numbers. Excessive weight was a problem. It took the wars of Korea and Vietnam to produce protective vests for common use, largely through the development of lightweight plastics such as Kevlar. They answered the need for an acceptable material of various weights and flexibilities, which still allowed for mobility and comfort. However, they couldn't protect all exposed body areas.

It is of historic interest that at the time that the Japanese surrendered on 15 August 1945, they already had plans to construct an armoured vest to protect a large area of the front of the chest and abdomen. At Milne Bay in September 1942, allied troops discovered an armour-plated jacket in the jungle. It was ingeniously composed of metal plates stitched into canvas pockets of a garment which weighed about five pounds. In its resistance to machine-gun and pistol fire, it was superior to any US vest being developed at that time. Much better designs became available in the Korean War, but undoubtedly the currently popular Kevlar jackets have improved greatly on the Japanese vests of the Second World War.

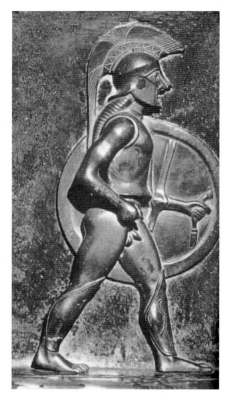

Lightweight Greek armour. The increasing level of protection over the centuries meant greater immobility. (*Unknown origin*)

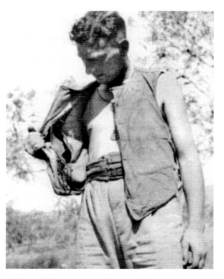

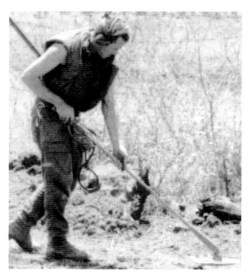

Above left: A Second World War Australian soldier demonstrates a Japanese bullet-proof vest found in New Guinea. Protective plates were fitted into internal slots. (*Unknown origin*)

Above right: A bomb-disposal engineer's inadequate protection, Second World War. (*Unknown origin*)

Today's armour is worn not only by military personnel but also by police, civilians in fear of assassination, and by some security staff. Although body-armour, goggles and a helmet provide a major survival advantage in modern warfare, areas of critical anatomic complexity, such as the eyes, face, neck, armpits and groins remain vulnerable. As surgeons see every day in combat zones, mines, improvised explosive devices and 'cluster' bombs still produce massive blast destruction of all limbs, particularly the legs. This global 'commotional' injury cannot be reduced significantly by any armour presently available or proposed.

The men who make safe the IEDs of modern warfare wear armoured suits that are reminiscent of space suits. They can reduce blast damage significantly, but not prevent it. Whereas the majority of 'clean' bullet wounds occur where the missiles actually enter and exit from the body, shrapnel usually stops just where it is meant to – deep inside the victim. Because of its jagged shape and fragmentation, survivors are often inflicted with extensive destruction of limbs and mutilation of the head and neck. They are the hallmark injuries of the young casualties who continue to flood army hospitals. Surgeons get little satisfaction from their remarkable salvage of those stunted bodies and lives, but such costs have become the standard currency of modern warfare.

'Just how well does body-armour really protect the wearer from firearm injuries?' is a question that Kobi Peleg and his surgical colleagues from Israel have asked themselves. They compared the effects of high-velocity missiles on soldiers who were 'protected' to some extent by their garments, and those of civilians who were completely 'unprotected'. 'Protection' meant wearing Kevlar, plastic-fibre vests with or without ceramic inserts, as well as military helmets. Of 669 terrorist injuries studied, about 40 per cent occurred in 'protected' soldiers and 60 per cent were in 'unprotected' civilians. Peleg was left in no doubt that mortality, the severity of injury, and the need for intensive care were all significantly greater in the unprotected victim.

As a result, all military persons and civilians outside the various forms of 'Green Zones' are ordered to wear protective helmets and vests whenever exposed to risk. Wearing the gear meant that troops who were fortunate enough to get to hospital care usually survived. With the 'unprotected', deaths occurred rapidly – usually within 24 hours of injury. Brain injury was significantly more common among unprotected civilians who rarely wore helmets, even if they wore vests. Apart from that aspect, the unprotected were also much more prone to widely spread injuries.

All Kevlar vests, and particularly those with inserted plates of metal, ceramic or polyethylene, protect the wearer by deflecting or absorbing the penetration and momentum of missiles into central body areas. While a helmet improves 'raw' survival, a reinforced vest protects the much larger areas of chest and abdomen. As expected, head injuries were likely to be more permanently limiting while abdominal and chest injuries, though more deadly, were at least potentially curable.

CHAPTER 6

Crimean War Catastrophe

I will have your arm off before you know where you are! The smart of the knife [without anaesthetic] is a powerful stimulant and it is better to hear a man bawl lustily than to see him sink silently into his grave.

– Sir John Hall, Crimea, 1854, The Wellcome Trust Centre

The Crimean War in Russia carried the highest mortality rate of all wars of the nineteenth and twentieth centuries. French and British forces were under the command of Lord Raglan, of whom Florence Nightingale said, '… wasn't a very great general, but … a very good man'. Despite the origins of the conflict, the ultimate players were the combined armies of Britain and France pitted against Russia.

Despite George Bernard Shaw's iconoclastic 1906 comment that 'Chloroform has done a lot of mischief. It's enabled every fool to be a surgeon,' he was never subjected to the appalling misery of a surgical procedure without general anaesthesia. Just as chloroform was becoming accepted, the Director-General of the Armed Medical Services of England had vetoed its use at Crimea. It demanded more care in its use than ether, but chloroform was non-flammable and in better supply. The Director-General found ether acceptable, but his reluctance to use chloroform was probably based on an ignorance of its advantages. As a result, his orders were considered to be uninformed and inhumane to such an extent that they were frequently disregarded.

Apocryphal or not, it is widely alleged that before general anaesthesia had become generally accepted, British surgeons in the Crimea conducted a competition to decide which of them could perform the quickest thigh amputation on a loudly complaining, un-anaesthetised patient. In his haste, the winner, with a two-minute procedure, inadvertently amputated the patient's genitals as well as his leg, two fingers of an assistant and the coat-tail of an onlooker. His victory was exceedingly hollow when the patient died from infection, the observer died from shock and the assistant died from septicaemia. He had, therefore, killed three people with one operation and, while his victims passed quickly into oblivion, his reputation for express surgery stood for all time. Whether or not the story is true, such conditions were common at Crimea before Florence Nightingale and her supporters changed all the old rules.

LADY OF THE LAMP

It may seem a strange principle to enunciate as the very first requirement in a hospital, that it should do the sick no harm ... a nurse should be ... devoted and obedient. This definition would do just as well for a porter. It might even be for a horse [but] it would not do for a policeman.

– Florence Nightingale, 1859

Florence Nightingale was born into a well-to-do British family living in Florence – from where she got her name. Early in life, she became inspired by the 'divine calling' of nursing, which had previously been a career of low reputation performed by poor women, camp-followers and cooks. She described the nurses whom she first encountered in London as being 'too old, too weak, too drunk, too dirty, too stolid and too bad to do anything else'. She applied a similar description to many British Army doctors and, in many respects, achieved much more than the medical profession did collectively in the latter half of the nineteenth century.

Against her family's wishes, she entered nursing in 1845 and, in effect, never left it. Her greatest contributions came in the reform of the Poor Laws, the establishment of a Sanitary Commission and Colleges of Nursing in Britain,

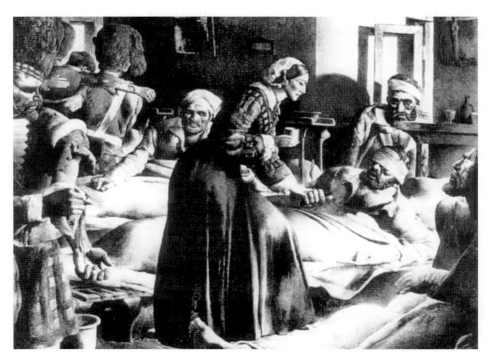

Depiction of Florence Nightingale in Crimea, assisting the injured. (*Wikipedia*)

and as a medical statistician. Originally representing 'The Institute for the Care of Sick Gentle Women in Distressed Circumstances', she persuaded her political friends to let her and her trainees go to Turkey. She championed the use of chloroform as a general anaesthetic and, after a short period of opposition, had little difficulty in persuading her medical colleagues to adopt its use generally.

In October 1854, she and thirty-eight volunteer nurses travelled to Scutari (in modern-day Istanbul) to assist overworked medical staff and to improve the appalling conditions for the wounded. Such an assignment had never before occurred. Ten times more soldiers were dying from infective diseases than from battle wounds; hospitals were vastly overfilled; sewers and ventilation systems were broken, blocked or non-existent; and general living conditions were primitive and filthy.

By dint of her persistence and powerful connections, she rapidly began to reverse the situation in Crimea. She was supported faithfully by Sydney Herbert, British Secretary of War and a man of great influence. He was so helpful that it was widely suspected that they were lovers. Whether or not that unlikely theory was true, she certainly became his key adviser and lifelong friend. She had several other lavish and persistent suitors but repelled them all. The given reason was that she wanted nothing to interfere with her calling to the noble art of nursing, which she regarded as God's work.

Nightingale returned from Crimea in 1857 amid rumours of a 'mental breakdown' from what might today be called a 'bipolar disorder', quite possibly a rumour to discredit her. She had made many enemies along her way. Without reference to any identified person and with no known treatment for whatever condition she had, she took up permanent accommodation at the Burlington Hotel in Piccadilly, where she isolated herself physically for most of the rest of her life. She did not, however, withdraw at all from public affairs and, from her room, she promoted the establishment of a Royal Commission on the Health of the army and wrote many detailed reports with her own expert statistical comment. She was rewarded with a major review of military surgery and the establishment of an Army Medical School with detailed medical records. She inaugurated nursing training at several London hospitals and published many notes on nursing procedures. In 1862, she became an honorary consultant to the Union government of the United States during the American Civil War. Reconciliation with her family never happened and, after her death, they rejected a government offer of a state funeral and burial in Westminster Abbey.

Whether or not she was an abrasive, self-confessed lesbian who came home from Scutari to stay in bed for fifty years, she was a politically aware and very effective protagonist for better conditions for doctors, nurses and fighting men.

Hilaire McCoubrey of Nottingham University has recounted the experience of Dr Edward Wrench, a British surgeon in charge of an army hospital in the

Russian Military Academy in Balaclava. Wrench saw the same horrors that had appalled Nightingale at Scutari – the inefficient treatment of the wounded and sick, the revolting physical conditions in which men lived and fought and an army bureaucracy paralysed by conflict. A colleague told Wrench that he had

> ... charge of 20 to 30 patients wounded from Inkerman, mixed with cases of cholera, dysentery and fever. There were no beds, or proper bedding. The patients lay in their clothes on the floor, which from rain blown in from the open windows and the traffic to and from the open-air latrines, was as muddy as a country road.

Modern concepts of sanitation didn't exist. In a letter written to his parents in 1854, Wrench could scarcely contain his revulsion:

> He [an un-named surgeon] is disgusted with everything and wants to go back to Scutari. He had the care of the Russian wounded. They had 130 last week but they have all died but sixteen. Our wounded are pretty well for [being] out here but [much] worse than the worst in any hospital in England. We have got no opium [for pain relief], arrow-root, tea or many other things, which of course does not facilitate the treatment. Wounds were infected by the heat and dust, by shortage of water and lack of proper care, and grew more and more painful. Foul exhalations contaminated the air, in spite of the praiseworthy attempts of the authorities to keep hospital areas in a sanitary condition. We were practically without medicines, the supply landed at the commencement of the campaign was exhausted and the reserve had gone to the bottom of the sea in the wreck of *The Prince*, so that in November 1854 even the base hospitals at Balaclava were devoid of opium, quinine, ammonia and, indeed, of all important drugs.

There seems no doubt that conditions in the hospitals at Balaclava and Sevastopol were medically indefensible by any standards of that time and would now also be legally indefensible as Wrench saw them:

> Things are in an awful state up here now and the patients, poor fellows, suffer dreadfully. I have just been round my wards for the night and have two men I don't expect to find alive in the morning. They are literally dying from exhaustion and we have nothing to give them. They are suffering from fever, like many more. We have not got a drop of wine to give them although there is lots at Balaclava. We have no means of getting it out.

In battlefield surgery involving amputations and other major interventions, an official directive that chloroform should *not* be used as an anaesthetic was regarded by Wrench as unacceptable. He didn't mince his words in reporting to his superiors:

> The cries of a patient undergoing an operation were satisfactory to the surgeon [only] as an indication that there was no fear of syncope and that the pain was a sting that aided recovery ... I have got a splendid case under my care just now. A man was hit in the arm three or four weeks ago. About two inches of ulna [forearm bone] was carried away and the bullet went clean through his arm. He was apparently doing well when frightful arterial haemorrhage set in one day when I was out of the camp. A surgeon plugged the wound and put a tourniquet on. This stopped it and, for another week, he did admirably. Then on Thursday last it bled again. I asked my senior surgeon's advice and he again recommended [the same treatment]. This stopped it but the wound had such an unhealthy appearance the next morning, that amputation was the only alternative. I therefore amputated his arm just above the elbow [without anaesthesia] and he is now doing admirably. No arm [at all] is much better for a soldier than an arm of little use ... for the first he gets a shilling a day pension [for the loss of the limb], whereas [with a useless – but attached – limb] he gets nothing but is just turned out as unfit for service ... the old story of, "when in doubt, operate", is doubly applicable in the army.

Given the longstanding decay of standards of military medicine in the British Army in the middle of the nineteenth century, the horrors experienced by Wrench were not altogether surprising. They were so bad that the original Geneva Convention of 1864 specifically criticised a war like the Crimean where resources were overwhelmed by the number of injured and transportation facilities were virtually absent. The wounded were left to wait on the pier at Balaclava for a ship to transport them out of their nightmare but there were few men who ever got away:

> The wretched patients [had been] jolted and tossed about by the mules on the mountain paths, the short road to Balaclava being then considered unsafe. Several mules fell and one poor soldier, recovering from a bullet through his chest, was thrown out and crimsoned the snow from his reopened wound. Poor Miss Nightingale was landed today at 4 o'clock and carried up to the convalescent hospital at Balaclava on a stretcher. She has got fever. I hope she will get better. She has been the saving of many lives herself. I am disgusted with anyone speaking ill of her. They little know what she has gone through. The big surgeons may call her interfering but the adjutants stick up for her and, as they were the men that did all the work at Scutari, they ought to know best.

It was the system and not the men that failed. The medical department was, like every other in the army of that day, quite unprepared for a great and prolonged war, hampered by red tape and denied all independence of action. The Crimean campaign taught a lesson I trust will never be forgotten, that unless the medical department of the army is made efficient and supplied with its proper complement of officers and ambulances during peace, it cannot be expected to do its duty efficiently during war.

Wrench gave great credit for improvements to Dr Henry Dunant, founder of the International Committee of the Red Cross (ICRC). Dunant had observed the Battle of Solferino in Italy in 1859, where 40,000 injured, dying and dead lay on the battlefield at the end of the day with no apparent attempt to help them.

The 1864 Geneva Convention was based on Dunant's reports for which he received the first Nobel Peace Prize in 1901. Wrench could well have qualified for another. Dunant's reports on the British Army supported those of Wrench and Nightingale. Between them, they ensured that the urgent need for effective international humanitarian law was finally appreciated and reforms began.

CHAPTER 7

American Civil War – The Dawn of Modern Surgery

I had a small group of cavalry with a couple of surgeons on a ridge blocking the path to my main base. The enemy sent a small wave of infantry up the hill. I charged and sabred them all down. My surgeon patched up [my men] in time to help me fight off the next large wave. By the third wave I had an army almost twice his size. I am a big believer in having a surgeon or two nearby.

– American Civil War Commander, 1862

Between 1861 and 1865, the very un-United States of America became involved in a violent civil war, probably the most important single event in US history. It happened during a period often regarded as the 'Middle Ages' of American surgery and its frenzy of mass destruction has never been matched before or since. The total mortality of that war – 600,000 dead – exceeded that of all others in which America has fought. About 40,000 of them were Negroes. Most died from a 'disease' of some sort, rather than from battle injury. A soldier had a one-in-three chance of surviving a term of combat duty.

It didn't help that the average soldier was almost impossible to command because he was a uniformed civilian with little or no war training. He lacked discipline and had poor morale and little confidence in the quality of his doctors. He knew that a significant limb injury, especially in the early stages of the war, would almost certainly bring an amputation without general anaesthesia.

Nothing much was known about what caused disease, how to stop it spreading or how to cure it. Too little had been learned from wars elsewhere or had never been known in North America with its geographic and cultural isolation from Europe. Surgical techniques were barbaric and often inept experiments. Harvard University owned only one stethoscope and one microscope during those war years. While most army doctors were, for the first time in the United States, called 'surgeons', their medical training was minimal compared with European medical schools. The war began with only 130 medical officers registered in the United States, but great surgical advances occurred before the war ended, largely because of the troubled consciences of exhausted surgeons and the endless complaints of anguished widows on both sides.

Four years later, 20,000 doctors were in war service, assisted by thousands of nurses who had willingly donated their time to help the wounded. The enormous numbers of casualties had moved many women to volunteer for duties that had once been despised as 'unladylike'. Indeed, one enterprising group of women's aid societies converted a Mississippi River steamer into a hospital ship, which saved thousands of lives. By the end of the war, 6,000 women had served in the Union Army alone and, for the first time in US history, ambulance services were plentiful and efficient. Although many Civil War doctors were regarded as 'butchers' by their patients and by the media, they did manage to treat more than 10 million injuries and illnesses within a two-year period of the war. A particular problem was the dreaded 'Minié' musket ball that produced huge, exploded wounds. So terrible were their effects that injuries of the head and abdomen were uniformly fatal and 20 per cent of all limb wounds required immediate amputation.

Primary care of the wounded was usually performed close to the battle lines and the survivors, with or without their amputations, were then taken by cart or wagon to field hospitals for convalescence. Because of the conditions under which they were forced to work, surgeons and nurses became increasingly strident in their complaints to all who would listen.

Towards the end of the war, chloroform anaesthesia had become available but a nurse of the time was still able to report a scene of total horror:

Screams that were heard were usually from soldiers just informed that they would lose a limb, or who were witness to the spectacle of other soldiers having operations. Tables about breast high had been erected upon which the screaming victims were having legs and arms cut off. The surgeons and their assistants, stripped to the waist and bespattered with blood, stood around,

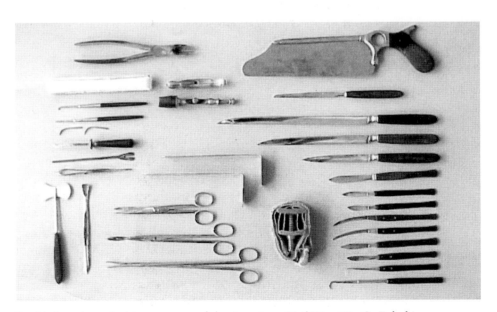

Sophisticated surgical instruments of the American Civil War. (*Dr G. Echols*)

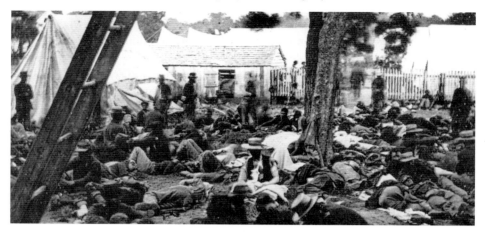

A confused view of a field dressing station, American Civil War. Few, if any, medical attendants are seen. (*US National Archives*)

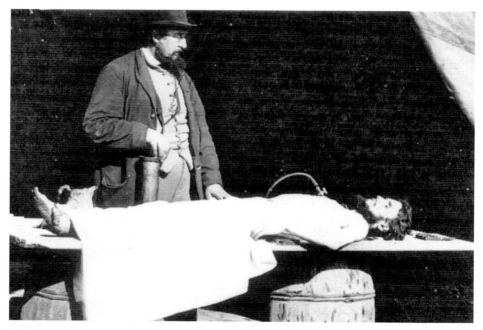

Failed surgery: an embalmer at work to enable repatriation of the corpse. (*Dr G. Echols*)

some holding the poor fellows while others, armed with long bloody knives and saws, cut and sawed away with frightful rapidity, throwing mangled limbs onto a pile nearby.

Most soldiers who died on both sides did so from non-combat disease. Men who were physically unfit before they joined the army, or were discovered to be so while in service, were easy prey to intestinal infections, pneumonia, tuberculosis and the common infectious diseases of civilian life. Typhoid fever and malaria spread uncontrollably. Pneumonia was often a fatal complication of even a simple cold. With camps littered with manure, offal and infected human waste, life was a dangerous misery for troops and their doctors alike.

Those who survived operations ran a great risk of wound infection. Surgeons clearly realised that there was a relationship between cleanliness and infection, but the bacterial nature of that connection escaped them for a long time. Among the many reasons for later improvements was an increasing trans-Atlantic flow of information from the Old World, including the teaching of principles of hygiene developed by Florence Nightingale and her London nurses.

However badly it had started, the Civil War finally heralded modern ideas of medicine and surgery into the United States and anaesthetists slowly became more competent with chloroform. Academically-minded surgeons sent thousands of amputated limbs to medical schools as specimens for both anatomy and war-wound teaching.

Ecumenically, by the end of 1863 most of the wounded from both sides were being treated at Letterman Hospital, named after Dr Jonathan Letterman, Medical Director of the Army of the Potomac River, and the dead were buried side by side in common cemeteries.

In 1863, Dr Letterman was moved to defend surgeons on both sides of the war:

The surgery of these battlefields has been called butchery ... a gross misrepresentation. To say so is to magnify an evil until it is beyond the

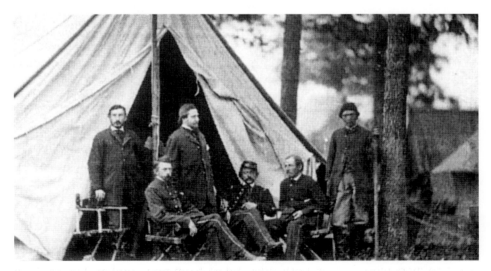

A surgical group relaxing. Dr Jonathan Letterman of Potomac is seated second from left. (*Dr G. Echols*)

bounds of truth. If there were any objection, it would be that the ethics on the part of surgeons to practice 'conservative surgery' were too great ... [in one case] the surgeons had been labouring since the battle to save the leg but it was impossible. The patient, a delicate-looking man, was put [partly] under the influence of chloroform and the amputation was performed with great skill by a surgeon who appeared to be quite accustomed to the use of his instruments. After the arteries were tied, the amputator scraped the end and edge of the bone until they were smooth. While the scraping was going on an attendant asked the patient, "How do you feel Corporal Thompson?" "Awful!," was the distinct and emphatic reply.

Letterman was among the many who deplored the catastrophic effects of the Minié bullet. He also insisted that surgeons should not continue to operate in bloody clothes without observing sterility just because they didn't believe in it or knew no better. They had to be taught the surgical rules regardless of ignorance of the reasons why – with their unclean stitches of horsehair, silk, cotton or linen, and without antibiotics or aseptic techniques – the ravages of septicaemia, gas gangrene and tetanus continued to account for 90 per cent of all deaths from wounding.

The 12 July 1862 edition of *Harper's Weekly* published a vignette of those times:

Away in the rear under the green flag which is always respected among civilised soldiers, the surgeon and his assistants received the poor wounded soldiers and swiftly administered to their needs. Arteries were tied, ligatures and tourniquets applied, flesh wounds hastily dressed, broken limbs set and sometimes, where haste was essential, amputations performed within sight and sound of the cannon. Of all officers, the surgeon is often the one who requires most nerve and most courage. The swaying tide of battle frequently makes him a prisoner and, sometimes, brutal soldiers will take a shot at him as they pass by. Upon his coolness and judgement depend the lives of a large proportion of the wounded and if they [the wounded] fall into the enemy's hands, military rule requires that [the surgeon] should accompany them as a prisoner. An arrangement has lately been made between General Cobb of the Rebel Army, and Colonel Keys of the Army of the Potomac [to the effect that] surgeons are to be considered non-combatants and released from custody as soon as their wounded are [back] in the hands of their own surgeons.

Out of the agony of the war, improved management of wounds of the head, chest, spine and blood vessels was established. Hospitals were opening across the land and paid nurses were being recruited. It is a tragedy of history that it took another century for the American Civil War to begin to deliver Thomas Jefferson's high ideals of 'Life, Liberty, and the pursuit of Happiness' to all

Americans. Ten years later, Dr Henry Porter, who had survived the Civil War, wrote of another surgical experience in which he exploited lessons learned during that war. In 1876, he was at Little Bighorn in Montana with General Custer, who fought the Sioux Indians because they were endangering the movement and settlement of migrants streaming westward. Custer's men had been badly mauled and Porter was the only survivor of three surgeons contracted to the army. His surgical equipment was in a wooden chest carried on a mule, just as surgeons had done at Waterloo. One of his men wrote of him with admiration:

> A hospital at Bighorn was established in about as safe a place as possible, the blue canopy of heaven being the covering, sand being the operating boards. But the stout heart and the nervy [*sic*] skilful hands of Dr Porter were equal to the situation.

Porter treated sixty-eight wounded men of whom only six died. Remarkably, one of three with abdominal wounds had survived – an almost unknown outcome in those years. One man on horseback was struck by a bullet which passed straight through his belt and into his belly. He got back into his saddle and was again struck, this time in his thigh. Porter recorded his thoughts frankly, 'We knew that he was doomed to die. Therefore we went to him with offers to write to his mother. The soldier refused the offer but asked for his tobacco pouch from his saddle pocket. He survived the injury and was again on duty four years later.'

Another soldier had his elbow joint blown away with resulting severe haemorrhage and shock. He was described as having, 'survived under the combined influence of surgery, stimulants per anum and electricity applied by an

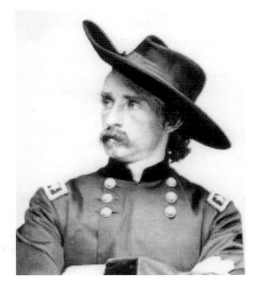

The legendary General George Custer of the American Civil War. (*Dr G. Echols*)

electric bath'. Such therapy had been prescribed in a medical text book of 1874 for the treatment of a wide array of conditions including paralysis, deafness, blindness, rheumatism and 'women's complaints'. Interestingly, Porter saw no cases of tetanus or gas gangrene in Montana, probably due to the dry climate and clean soil. Nor were there the usual reports of rattlesnake bites or arrow wounds in the survivors of Custer's battles. It was revealed much later that a few corpses had been 'mutilated' by the Indians, presumably by scalping.

RICH HARVEST

Dr Edward E. Hume has written extensively on the benefits to mankind of army medicine, largely predicated on the experience of the American Civil War, which led to the establishment of three great American institutions – the Army Medical Library, the Army Medical Museum and the Army Medical School. The Chief Surgeon of the army in the First World War described Dr Walter Reed's understanding of Yellow Fever, a massive killer, as revealing:

> … a secret of nature materially affecting the prosperity of nations, and the lives, fortunes and happiness of thousands [perhaps an underestimation]. Fewer still succeed in so quickly convincing brother scientists and men in authority of the truth of their discoveries.
>
> Armies promoted studies of nutrition, dentistry, psychiatry, hospital building and administration, infectious and parasitic diseases such as tuberculosis, cholera, dysentery, malaria, cholera, dengue fever, X-rays, nursing, physiotherapy and rehabilitation, aviation and naval medicine.

In 1888, Louis Pasteur, who had been the first to identify bacteria as the cause of infections in the same year as the start of the American Civil War, foretold with great insight the future of military medicine:

> Two opposing laws seem to be now in contest. The one law of blood and death, opening out each day new modes of destruction, forces nations to always be ready for battle. The other, a war of peace, work and health, whose only aim is to save a man from the calamities which beset him. The one seeks violent conquests, the other the relief of mankind. The one places a single life above victories, the other sacrifices hundreds of thousands of lives. The law of which we are the instruments strives even through the carnage to cure wounds due to the law of war. Treatment by our antiseptic methods may preserve the life of thousands of soldiers. Which of these two laws will prevail, only God knows. But of this we may be sure – with science and obeying the laws of humanity, we will always labour to enlarge the frontiers of life.

CHAPTER 8

War Against Politicians

I will smash the CIA into a thousand pieces.

– President John Kennedy after the failed CIA attempt to wrest government from Fidel Castro, April 1961

The Warren Commission! What the hell would they know? Did they learn anything you couldn't read in the papers the next day?

– Jack Ruby, letter quoted in *Argosy* magazine, September 1967

The inventors of our history are forever fetched by that lone, mad killer, eaten up with resentment and envy, the two principal American emotions, if our chroniclers are to be believed. Yet the gunning down in public view with his wife to one side and all the panoply of state fore and aft is pure Palermo send-off.

– Gore Vidal, *The Last Empire: Essays 1992–2000*

The assassinations of four American Presidents and the brother of one of them were forerunners of today's terrorist wars. It is unrewarding to quibble about whether they were acts of terrorism or anarchy. Their reasons and effects were exactly the same but with a different sort of war and different surgeons.

Impossible demands were placed on doctors who suddenly found themselves managing catastrophic events involving a president at the scene of their occurrence. Of course, surgeons who became involved were placed in highly visible positions of extreme difficulty. It is informative to examine how they handled those challenges and with what degree of success – what any surgeon could, or could not possibly accomplish in those circumstances becomes very obvious.

Assassins employed stealth, premeditation and dedication and all must have known that they were liable to capture and severe retribution soon after they had carried out their missions. They exhibited many characteristics of modern 'suicide bombers' – each was driven by an absolute conviction of the merit of exterminating a public figure. Despite many conspiracy theories, all but one of those blamed seemed to have acted in isolation. Three of the five victims, Lincoln and both Kennedys, died from massive injuries to the head with no real chance of recovery.

With no antibiotics available, even the most skilled surgery of the time would probably have failed with the abdominal injuries of Garfield and McKinley. While they may have been saved by expert modern care, that possibility becomes irrelevant when the nature of their wounds and the available surgical resources of the time are taken into consideration. Due to the particular circumstances of each attack, the initial resuscitation and surgical attention the victims received were probably inadequate or useless in every case. All of the assassins had political or quasi-political intent and all of them were experienced with weapons. At the same time, every victim was well aware of security needs and their own vulnerability. Three of the presidents had lived through the Civil War and knew of its social implications.

Abraham Lincoln had been the target of numerous death threats from Southerners who didn't want slavery abolished. John Booth was familiar with the theatre and a popular enough actor to command an income similar to that of Lincoln. In the interests of preserving slavery, he conspired with others to kill Lincoln, the Vice President, the Secretary of State, the Secretary of War and General Ulysses Grant when the opportunity presented. During an evening performance at Ford's Theatre in Washington DC, Booth shot Lincoln through the back of the head, having chosen a moment during a play when he could approach the president without much difficulty. He left the theatre by vaulting

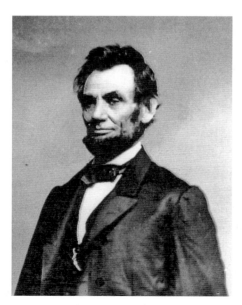

President Abraham Lincoln, 1809–1865. (*Wikipedia*)

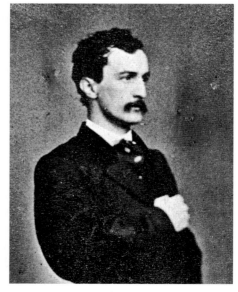

John Wilkes Booth, Lincoln's killer. (*The Library of Congress*)

over the rail of the box onto the stage in front of a stunned audience. Despite fracturing his left fibula, he fled to a waiting horse but later needed surgical attention by Dr Samuel Mudd, who gave assistance without telling anybody what he had done.

The first doctor on the scene was a 24-year-old army surgeon, Charles Leale. He instituted first-aid measures of some sort and attempted to open the scalp wound with his finger to remove clots in the hope that it would relieve pressure on Lincoln's brain. Three other doctors soon arrived on the scene and repeatedly probed the wound with bare fingers (there were no surgical gloves in those days) to try to find the bullet. Lincoln rapidly became moribund and died early the next morning. An autopsy performed in the White House showed that the bullet had passed from behind Lincoln's left ear to the front of his brain. It has recently been suggested that he might have survived that injury with more aggressive surgical care, but that is unlikely in view of the extent of the injury and the inevitable amount of reactionary brain swelling. If, miraculously, he had initially survived – or if he survived today with modern treatment – it is certain that Lincoln would have been vegetative at best. All attending physicians probably acted reasonably, but what they did to the wound with their bare fingers was scarcely ideal practice. In the end, they did not affect the outcome because they could not have produced useful relief of compression of the haemorrhaging brain.

Booth had fancied himself as a killer of tyrants. His motives were quite simple but it was pure political murder. When finally cornered, he was given several opportunities to surrender peacefully but rejected them all and was shot through the neck by Sergeant Thomas Corbett. The wound defied any contemporary surgical care and he suffocated on the porch of a Virginia farmhouse as a result of a spinal injury.

James Garfield was shot on 2 July 1881 by Charles Guiteau, who believed that the President favoured another Civil War. Guiteau was convinced that he had God's approval to assassinate Garfield who was in Washington on his way to a college reunion. The killer approached from behind and fired two shots into Garfield's back. One wound was superficial and did no real harm but the other took a complicated course through several upper abdominal organs. First on the scene was Dr Smith Townsend, the district health officer, who probed the major back wound thoroughly with his unwashed finger (again before rubber gloves were invented), hoping to find the bullet, but he failed to do so. The President was then transferred to the White House in a shocked state. At his own request, he was placed in the care of a Dr Bliss.

Some hours later a naval surgeon, Dr Wales, also examined the wound with his bare fingers and concluded that the bullet had passed through the liver and lay in the abdominal cavity somewhere. Half a dozen other curious doctors repeated the performance and nodded their heads wisely, no doubt, but none of them was able to find the bullet with a finger. At least two of them

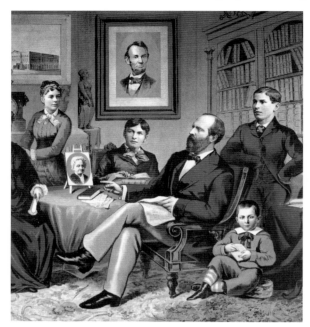

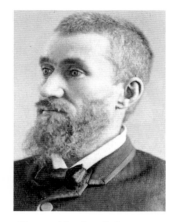

Above: Charles Guiteau, 1841–1882. (*Wikipedia*)

Left: President James Garfield with some members of his family, 1831–1881. (*Library of Congress*)

were highly experienced surgeons. Why they wanted to know where the bullet was, rather than what damage it had produced, is unclear. It seems that no exploratory operation was planned.

For a couple of months, Garfield slowly improved. During that period, Alexander Graham Bell, the Scottish inventor of the telephone, offered to construct a machine which might locate the bullet by an auditory reflection-signal, presumably an early form of ultra-sound. Finally, Bell gave up despite many tests and was forced to withdraw, probably gratefully, when the President suddenly deteriorated. With increasing evidence of deep infection in his chest and in his abdomen, he suddenly died. Autopsy showed pockets of pus and massive haemorrhage around a ruptured artery.

Guiteau was hanged nine months later, insisting that God had told him to kill Garfield. All the doctors who attended Garfield submitted huge accounts to the US government and all were promptly paid in full. A half-hearted enquiry into the size of the accounts was suddenly aborted by order of the succeeding President. As with Lincoln, it is widely agreed that repeated, unhygienic examination of Garfield's wound could well have introduced a mortal infection, but, in any case, it is unlikely that he could have survived his wounds. Nobody was anxious to undertake an exploratory operation on a President who seemed to be improving. He certainly had no expert nursing care, but that would scarcely have hastened his death. Clearly, his management failed to meet ideal standards, but it did not affect the outcome.

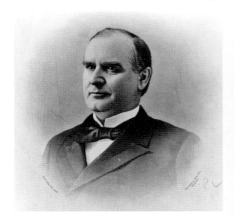

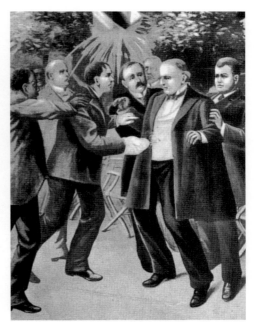

Above: President William McKinley,
1843–1901. (*Wikipedia*)

Right: Depiction of the attack on
William McKinley by Leon Czolgosz.
(*Wikipedia*)

Organised global terrorist activities were clearly apparent in that era. Three months before Garfield died, Tsar Alexander II of Russia was killed by a hand grenade thrown by an anarchist. As well as these two men, in the following twenty years anarchists also killed the President of France, the Empress of Austria and the King of Italy. During the investigation of the King's death in 1898, a note was found naming six world leaders whom anarchists planned to kill. The first three on the list were already dead.

The fifth was President William McKinley. Like Garfield, President William McKinley had a distinguished record during the Civil War and was believed to be popular. Because Leon Czolgosz was dedicated to world anarchy, he shot the President twice on 4 September 1901, in Buffalo City, New York. There was a superficial injury to the right upper chest and a deep wound of the upper abdomen. Quickly on the scene was a Dr George Hall, accompanied by two medical students. They saw much external bleeding and took the President to a nearby hospital which was ill-equipped to handle any surgical emergency. Other surgeons soon arrived, some of them experienced in gunshot wounds during the Civil War. For some reason, they decided unanimously that Dr Matthew Mann, an obstetrician and gynaecologist, should be in charge of surgical management. There may have been some conflict of opinion among the various surgeons present about that choice but it transpired that the least appropriate surgeon ended up as the leader of the team of operators. With inadequate instruments, poor lighting and unhelpful assistance, exploration of the President's upper abdomen showed a large tear of the stomach.

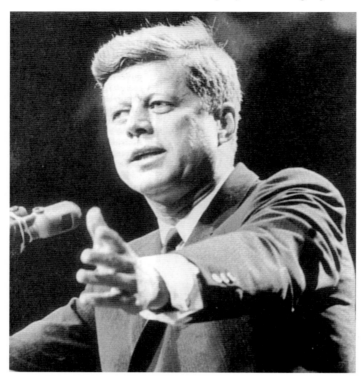

President John
F. Kennedy, 1917–
1963. (*Wikipedia*)

By that date, rubber gloves were available and reasonable sterility was possible, but there was already much soiling of the cavity by spilled stomach contents. Some reports referred to other injuries of the colon and kidney, but no mention was made of surgical attention to those organs. Because of the nature of the wound, it is unlikely that the availability of antibiotics could have contributed favourably to the outcome. Dr Mann repaired the stomach and the President was taken to a nearby house for convalescence. No fewer than eight experienced nurses were allocated to McKinley's care – such an over-abundance being related, perhaps, to the quite inadequate nursing of President Garfield.

The intensive care given was appropriate to 1901 and included adrenalin, oxygen, nutrient enemas of egg and whiskey, and water, camphor and nitro-glycerine by mouth. The surgeons agreed to McKinley's request for cigars before he abruptly died on the eighth day after his operation. An autopsy showed extensive infection in all the upper abdominal organs.

It was generally agreed that surgical management was undertaken in an inappropriate place by an inappropriate surgeon with multiple assistants who were of doubtful help to the surgeon. Whether or not the injuries to the colon and kidney affected the outcome, it seems that Dr Mann had been handed a poisoned chalice, perhaps because nobody wanted the responsibility

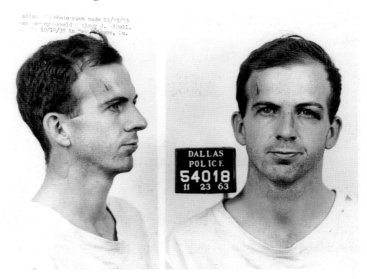

Lee Harvey
Oswald, 1939–
1963.

for managing the President's wounds. Again, all practitioners involved in McKinley's care submitted extravagant accounts, which were paid in full but without haste. Czolgosz was executed a month after the shooting.

John Kennedy opposed Communism while Lee Harvey Oswald embraced the form practised by Castro in Cuba. Oswald had originally planned to kill President Richard Nixon but no opportunity had arisen. The usual interpretation of the situation is that, while working at the Texas School Book Depository in Dallas, Oswald learned that Kennedy was to visit the city and pass the Depository. He decided to kill him to demonstrate his dedication to Communism.

On 22 November 1963, Kennedy and his wife were in the back seat of an open car, moving slowly through the middle of a large crowd. Governor John Connally and his wife were sitting in front. It is now generally accepted that, at around noon, Oswald fired three shots from the sixth floor of the Depository. The first carbine bullet missed the group altogether. The second passed through Kennedy's neck and then struck Governor Connally. The third bullet struck the back of the President's head. He was taken to nearby Parkland Hospital within five minutes.

The first doctor involved was a surgical resident, Dr James Carrico, who found Kennedy in extremis with extruded brain tissue and heavy bleeding. Although appropriate resuscitative measures were applied and several specialists were soon available, Kennedy was pronounced dead thirty minutes after his injury. An autopsy showed massive, irrecoverable damage to the right half of his brain. There was also a deep wound on the right side of his neck which obstructed his airway.

Although Dr Carrico had noted both entry wounds, the neck injury was not originally identified by the Parkland Hospital staff but, despite that oversight, nothing could have saved Kennedy's life. Governor Connally recovered from his multiple injuries.

Shortly after the President was attacked, Oswald shot and killed a policeman who attempted to capture him. He was arrested shortly after in a movie theatre. Two days later, in the busiest part of a Dallas police station, a nightclub owner, Jack Ruby, shot Oswald in the chest and he died during an exploratory operation.

A minor criminal with Mafia connections who often carried a handgun, Ruby's motive still remains unclear. He was apprehended after he had shot Oswald in what became the first-ever homicide on a live-to-air TV broadcast. Ruby was sentenced to death, but appealed and had a new trial pending when he died. John Kennedy, Oswald and Ruby all died in Parkland Hospital, Dallas.

Sirhan Sirhan attempted to assassinate Senator Robert Kennedy, the US Attorney General and brother of President John Kennedy, just after the Senator had won the Californian Presidential Primary on 5 June 1968.

Sirhan and many onlookers were in a crowded kitchen corridor through which Kennedy was leaving the Ambassador Hotel after addressing supporters. As he passed slowly through the pack, Sirhan fired into the crowd around the Senator. Several shots struck Kennedy, one hitting his clothing, one or two entering his right chest superficially and another striking his head.

The first doctor on the scene, Stanley Abo, found a wound behind Kennedy's right ear with a powder burn indicating a very close range shot from behind. He probed the wound with a bare finger in an attempt to allow free exit of

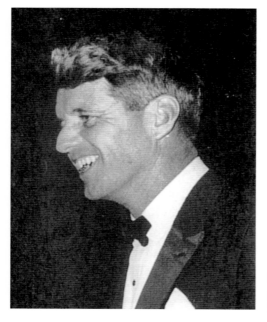

Senator Robert F. Kennedy, 1926–1968, possibly assassinated by Sirhan Sirhan. (*Wikipedia*)

blood and reduce the pressure of bleeding on Kennedy's brain before he was quickly transferred to the closest hospital.

With no neurosurgeon available there, he was then rushed to the Good Samaritan Hospital where surgeons found the other wounds – one in the right armpit and another a few inches below. During the operation, neurosurgeons removed blood clots and fragments of bullet and bone from Kennedy's shattered brain, but he died within twenty-four hours. Autopsy confirmed a huge injury to the right side of Kennedy's brain and brain stem, but the shots that struck the right side of his chest had not injured him mortally.

Sirhan had actually fired eight shots, some of which struck bystanders. Mystery surrounds the fact that an armed guard close behind Kennedy had also fired a shot, but his weapon was never checked by the police and the crime-scene photographs were destroyed or lost before Sirhan's trial.

The shot that killed Kennedy entered the back of his head and had been fired at almost point-blank range, but, according to all those interrogated, Sirhan had only fired from in front of Kennedy. Unless Kennedy had turned through almost 90 degrees at the instant he was shot – and there is no evidence for that – it is difficult to see how Sirhan's shot could have been responsible for Kennedy's mortal injury. It is even more difficult to see how the guard's shot could be disregarded as the fatal one. Not surprisingly, the autopsy pathologist's report was carefully worded:

> Until more is precisely known ... the existence of a second gunman remains a possibility. Thus, I have never said that Sirhan killed Robert Kennedy.

That comment begs several questions: did the security guard in fact fire the deadly shot? Was the shot deliberate? Who else might have wanted Kennedy dead? Was the guard aiming at Sirhan? Why were details and materials of the police enquiry hidden or lost? The enigma persists.

Sirhan confessed to the killing but then claimed no memory of the event. As with John Kennedy, conspiracy theories about Robert Kennedy's assassination remain unanswered. At Sirhan's trial, the question was repeatedly raised as to whether the shot which killed Kennedy had come from Sirhan's gun, but there was no confident answer. The security guard was cleared of involvement.

Given the wording of the autopsy report, Sirhan's original death sentence was commuted to life imprisonment. Since then, he has applied unsuccessfully for parole on at least thirteen occasions. In 2009, he was in a Californian State Prison with a further chance of parole in 2011. His diaries, though confused, repeatedly suggest that his reason for attacking Kennedy was the latter's support for Israel in the 1967 Six-Day War.

CHAPTER 9

The First World War, 1914–1918

A cry from No Man's Land cuts like a drill into our heads. We wither and grow old between those cries ... a man crying for assistance for three days when his stretcher bearers had been killed.

    – Ernest Toller, German Surgeon, 1914, Spartacus Educational

... the wretchedness of dying young men, faces turned to the wall, whimpering and calling for their mothers. We passed too many days hoping, waiting patiently and suffering together, hoping the fever would abate, scrutinising the wound and searching for the deep roots of decay, both [surgeon and patient] quaking.

    – John Kirkup, Curator, Royal College of Surgeons of England, 1914

Placed end-to-end, the trenches of the First World War would have encircled the Earth. Flowing a furtive power struggle in the Balkans in 1914, Austria, Hungary, Germany, Turkey and Bulgaria ultimately confronted Russia, Italy, Britain, Japan, France, Portugal, Romania, China and the United States. The First World War was fought on many fronts with massive casualties on both sides.

It is fair to say that medical and surgical services had deteriorated greatly in the largely battle-idle century before, and that none of the combatants were equipped to manage huge numbers of casualties. The war introduced for the first time the use of tanks, while the effects of artillery compounded the medical challenges on both sides.

British and American medicine had developed quite differently in the late nineteenth century, but ignorant bureaucracies in Britain had retarded developments that might have saved countless lives in the First World War. On the other hand, the American Civil War had raised standards to such an extent that, of 250,000 American wounded during the First World War, only 6 per cent died – only a marginally greater percentage than in the Second World War. For the Americans, at least, surgical innovations made war progressively less lethal at the price of leaving more disabled survivors to be rehabilitated.

The trenches became a nightmare – the outcome of the progression of Western Civilisation. Men under attack by shells, mortars and grenades had nowhere to go and surgical help was difficult to reach. There were too few anaesthetists available and their training had not kept pace with surgical developments. Wound infections by tetanus and gas gangrene were endemic in the trenches.

Most psychological casualties returned to some sort of duty after perfunctory treatment, but two-thirds of all British pensions were related to stress. Strangely, only a small number were awarded for gas inhalation, perhaps because many had died before their pensions had been approved.

Armies had about four stretcher-bearers for every 200 soldiers. For some reason, wounded men's colleagues were ordered not to treat them while they awaited expert evacuation to a first-aid post. As a result, hundreds of men died every day as they quietly waited for the assistance that never came. The persistently wet conditions of Europe made the job of stretcher-bearers and first-aid men almost impossible. It could take four hours to carry an injured man half a mile and, being upright and close together, helpers were easy targets even for erratic gunfire. The result was that thousands of men fought and died in quagmires of mud, sewage and decaying corpses beneath the menaces of bombing and gassing. Compounding their misery, sleep was almost impossible.

Although Lord Kitchener had banned journalists from the Western Front in 1914, one of them joined a Red Cross unit as a stretcher-bearer and reported

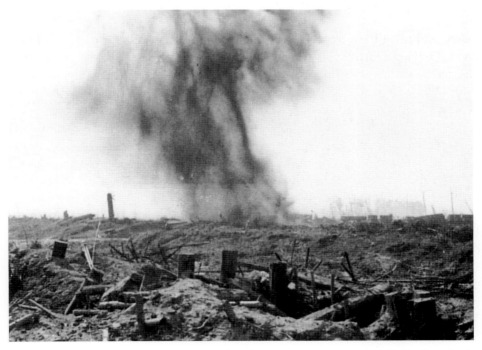

Constant barrage of shells and bombs caused devastating injuries and shell-shock on both sides in the First World War. (*R. Ruggenberg*)

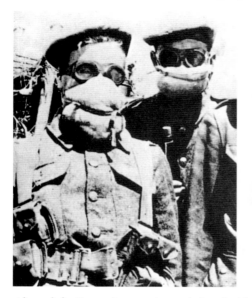 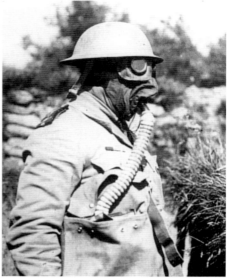

Above left: Protective goggles and chemical-loaded gas masks, 1915. (*R. Ruggenberg*)

Above right: More sophisticated filtering masks (possibly asbestos), Europe, 1917. (*R. Ruggenberg*)

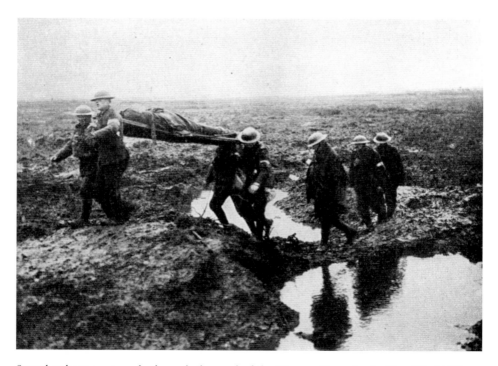

Stretcher-bearers struggle through the mud of the Western Front in the First World War. Progress was slow and dangerous from exposure to enemy fire.

on '… the bestiality, futility and insanity of a war when men were taught to kill, maim and mutilate each other, without any quarrel [existing] between them'.

The vulnerable No Man's Land on the Western Front measured about 250 metres in width, filled with barbed wire up to 30 metres deep; a long, narrow field scattered with bodies, pocked by shell craters filled with contaminated water and, by night, illuminated brilliantly by rockets and flares. In these conditions, men on both sides were expected to be vigilant, enthusiastic and prepared to risk exposure on patrols. With fixed bayonets, their value lay far more in intimidation than effectiveness. A distinguished Australian surgeon, Captain John Kirkup, concluded that it was almost impossible to manage trench injuries adequately before 1917.

To begin to bring rates of death, infection and amputation under some degree of control, increased numbers of stretcher-bearers were needed, as well as better splints for leg fractures, plentiful blood for transfusion, and faster evacuation of the wounded by motor ambulance. The rapid application of splints with traction to straighten and immobilise fractures became standard treatment for open thigh fractures, with a remarkable 70 per cent reduction of mortality, just by minimising the shock that could arise from the grating of fractured bone ends.

Bullets were the least common missile and they caused much less damage than shell, bomb, grenade or shrapnel injuries. Most shrapnel casualties had

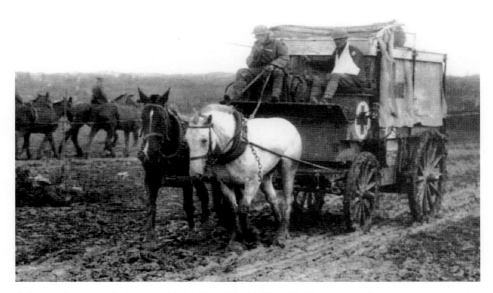

A horse-drawn ambulance vehicle, First World War. (*R. Ruggenberg*)

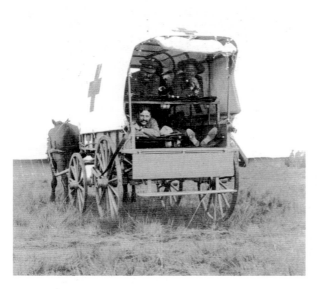

A First World War, double-decker, horse-drawn ambulance with patients sitting above and lying below. (*R. Ruggenberg*)

extensive soft tissue damage – contaminated foreign materials blasted deep into wounds made 'debridement' more difficult, but more urgent than ever before if gangrene, leading to amputation and death, was to be reduced.

Men with fractures of arms and some with less severe fractures of their shins could move alone or with help, but those with fractured thighs were immobilised and depended entirely on stretcher-bearers. At any one time, hundreds of wounded men on both sides lay alone for days without food or water in the shell holes of No Man's Land, waiting for help. One British soldier reported that he was saved by an injured German who had dragged himself into the same shell hole for protection. They shared the German's provisions and both survived.

If men were fortunate enough to be retrieved on stretchers, they could be taken no further than the open ground around casualty clearing stations to await transport to a better facility. For many, that never happened. A British war history described a familiar scene:

… stretcher-bearers struggling 4,000 yards carrying inert and badly stricken comrades across open plains or along muddy shell-swept trenches or roads … to reach some point where wheeled transport was available. They had to negotiate barbed wire and other obstacles, traverse steep trenches, often flooded or deep in mud, trying to avoid jolting the shocked patient. They could move more freely at night, even under flare light, than in broad daylight.

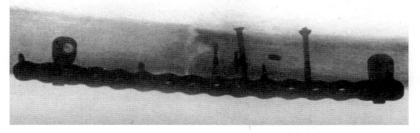

Unstable thigh fracture repositioned and fixed by metal plate and screws
– bone ends not fully approximated. (*Dr M. Crumplin*)

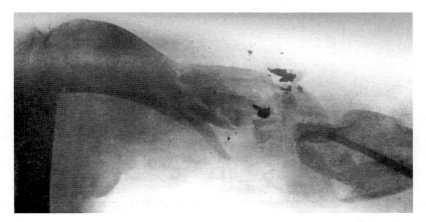

Shrapnel embedded in a shattered arm with such bone loss as to make
amputation necessary. (*Dr M. Crumplin*)

The injured had large doses of morphine before stretcher transportation. On
the Somme, all 34 stretcher-bearers of one battalion became casualties in one
morning, paralysing the recovery of troops generally.

The military historian, Sir John Keegan, concluded that, 'There were simply
too many casualties and too few doctors – too few anybodies.' The 'triage' or
sorting of wounded men into levels of priority couldn't work in and around
the trenches because so little could be done for most of the significantly
injured.

To further complicate matters, injured men who had been triaged into one of
the three major categories – trivial, treatable or terrible – needed reassessment
frequently enough to determine changes in their condition. That affected the
urgency of evacuation, the type of treatment required and the best place to
have it; but so little was possible that it became a futile, academic exercise or
gesture. It is recorded that the Germans offered British commanders short,
unofficial truces to allow their wounded to be retrieved on stretchers, but there
is no evidence that the British ever reciprocated the gesture.

The 'trivial' (walking-wounded) and the 'terrible' cases were easy problems. The former were patched up and returned to battle as soon as possible. The others were managed by generous doses of opium, reassurance and the merciful attention of padres. It was the middle group, the seriously injured but potentially salvageable cases who, as always, presented the greatest practical and ethical difficulties for surgeons when evacuation and first aid were slow or impossible. For the carers, a degree of compromise was inevitable.

Many injured men found themselves on the wrong side of a changing No Man's Land or even stranded within formal enemy positions and liable to be wounded again. Those with severe wounds of the chest and abdomen were little problem – tragically, they died quickly with or without medical attention. Shock killed relentlessly but there was little to be done for it unless it was suspected early and treated immediately by adequate blood transfusion – an impossibility in the early phases of the war.

According to military historians, injuries sustained on the Somme were much worse than had ever been seen at Waterloo. Deep impaction of foreign material and shrapnel into wounds usually led to gas gangrene and death. Bomb blasts could kill men and leave little external evidence of injury, while their lungs, bowels, ears, brains and spinal cords had been pulped. There are many accounts of men melting or disappearing when enveloped in the blast of a bursting shell. Many bayonet wounds seen in No Man's Land seemed to have been inflicted after death, either from spite or to be absolutely sure a man could participate no more.

The wounds of trench warfare were completely new and shocking to most surgeons. Early experience showed that immediate closure of wounds by stitching was disastrous because infected tissue was left inside to ferment and generate gangrene. Instead, wherever an anaesthetist was available, foreign bodies and dead tissue had to be thoroughly removed. Those wounds were then washed with antiseptics such as 'Milton', carbolic or iodine before being filled softly with 'Vaseline-gauze' packing, but no stitches were used until after evacuation.

Later decision-making concerned when and whether to close wounds. If they appeared clean and healing at the end of a week, some could safely be closed, at least partly, but many open (compound) limb fractures needed early amputation, however carefully they had been managed. The extent of muscle pulping and decay often became apparent only after days of regular observation. That required adequate notes of past treatment when a man reached his next point of evacuation.

Troops and field doctors knew little of where they were, where they were meant to be and in which direction to go. H. L. Smith was an ambulance officer who saw action at St Mihiel and reported that grossly infected wounds had been miraculously cleaned by maggot infestation, just as surgeons had described hundreds of years earlier. He described a particular afternoon when

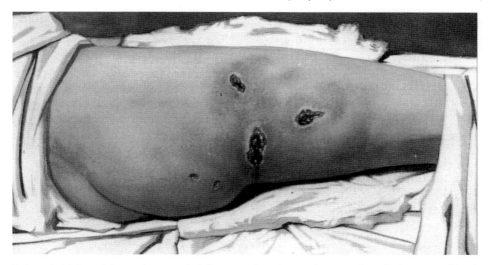

Infected thigh and buttock wounds left open after shrapnel removal to drain pus and heal slowly. (*Dr M. Crumplin*)

confusion was magnified by his group suddenly encountering half a million American troops and four French divisions operating from the concealment of forests alongside their position. Finding themselves ignored by that huge force and with no idea of its intentions, British surgeons, ambulance officers, nurses and stretcher-bearers of Smith's detachment just continued with their tasks: '… remote from the world, among a maelstrom of shells and bullets, shattering sky and earth, flaying gouts of mud and chalk into the air'.

At the end of one long day, Smith saw an Australian surgeon enter a tent where some of his colleagues were having a lavish dinner of confiscated food and wine. 'Why, you bastards!' he shouted. 'Don't ever sit down again to stuff your guts until you see that your men have been fed and watered properly. Now get the hell out of here until every man has been cared for!'

Before he went to war, Dr John Hayward had done some minor surgery at a local hospital in England, where he had been a general practitioner for twenty years. He had also experienced bigger surgery at a small Red Cross Hospital in the first six months of the war, but he knew little of the nature of cases fresh from the battlefield or of the surgical techniques to deal with them. His 1918 memoirs of a casualty clearing station in France describe a large base hospital at Trouville:

> … full of the wastage of war – men sent down from the Front suffering from the ordinary diseases of civil life which should have precluded their enlistment. The Front knocked them out almost at once and they came to [us to] be patched up, to convalesce and return. The mess was full of rather war-weary (medical) men who had endured much and were glad of an easy berth.

I had plenty of operating on ordinary civil life disabilities and, when not engaged with filling out forms, enjoyed myself in field expeditions to collect butterflies and flowers, but the distant sound of guns was often disturbing.

But another base hospital at Amiens was very different. There he found that military discipline, red tape and formality were minimal. The development of small mobile hospitals near the fighting line revolutionised the surgery of the war and saved thousands of lives. It was generally accepted that the fatal infection and gangrene of wounds were reduced only if effective operation could be performed within thirty-six hours of wounding. All debris and dead tissue had to be removed, regardless of the amount of mutilation involved. Those simple measures were the key to survival. Hayward described the essential parts of a casualty clearing station:

> It had a large reception tent, a side-tent for the moribund, another resuscitation tent for the severely injured to be resuscitated by warming and blood transfusion, another for preparation of cases for operation and a larger tent containing six operating tables completely equipped and staffed. From a recovery area, convalescent men were sent to await the hospital train while those who needed further observation, or were too ill to be evacuated, were retained for at least another day or so.
>
> I had two days to settle down and get some idea of my new surroundings and everyone was immensely kind, but I realised how entirely inexperienced I was in the work which would be required of me. My colleagues were all young men with two or three years war service. Vast reserves of men and transport have silently been moving up the road to Amiens to support the Australian attack at Villers-Bretonneux. On my third day I was orderly officer and then had to be on duty all night as reception officer.

On that evening, an enemy attack began in earnest with a continuous roar of heavy artillery, star shells and the flashes of exploding bombs. In the early morning, ambulances began to arrive at the clearing station. One after the other, the wounded were taken on stretchers or wearily stumbled into Hayward's tent, some fully clothed and others wrapped only in blankets or coats stiffened with dried blood, mud and dirt, bandaged or splinted and carrying labels of their injuries from the first-aid posts:

> They come in such numbers the tent is soon filled … I can't cope with them all … many of them are white and cold and lie still and make no response and those who do, are laconic or just point to their labels. I have had no instruction on how to dispose of such numbers or the method of procedure but I realised that they must be examined briefly and sorted and sent to one or other of our hospital tents.

But my orderly was at my side with whispered suggestions and soon we had the stretchers on one side and the standing cases on the other and, leaving the slighter cases to be dressed, I gradually sorted out the bad ones for resuscitation, pre-op, or evacuation tents. I had never seen such frightful wounds and could not conceive how we three surgeons could deal with them on the ensuing days.

Hayward and his colleagues often worked without interruption or relief for twenty-four or thirty-six hours and, during one such spell, he believed he was looking into Dante's hell:

In this charnel tent of pain and misery there was silence and no outward expression of moans or groans or complaints. The badly shocked had passed beyond it; others appeared numbed or too tired to complain or so exhausted that they slept as they stood. Even the badly wounded often asked for a smoke. Here were lying uncomplaining men with shattered heads or ghastly disfiguration of their faces, others with shell and bullet wounds to the chest, spitting blood and gasping for breath and, worst of all, those quiet, afraid-to-be-touched cases with an innocent tiny little mark where the bullet had entered (the belly) but already the thready pulse, drawn corners of the mouth, anxious look and rigid muscles which betoken hopeless disaster within.

He classified as 'multiple-wounded' one group of men similar to the patients called 'Balad Specials' seen in Baghdad today:

Their bodies [were] riddled with large or small shell fragments, [with] terrible compound fractures in Thomas splints and the stumps of torn off limbs. It began to take away all [my] self confidence. I began to think of the bad luck of the wretched victims who came under my knife. How confidently they went under the ether, relying on my skills; how their lives and the happiness of their homes depended upon me; how much better for them had fate brought them to the next surgical table. Every feeling and introspection that should never cross a surgeon's mind began to possess me and shake my nerve. Only concentration on the actual technique of the operation kept me going.

He wondered if the various tent wards would ever be emptied. The memory of the haunted faces of their inmates remained fixed in his mind forever. The resuscitation tent was the most dreadful place, filled with the shocked and collapsed and dying who were unfit to tolerate operations until warmed up in heated beds and transfused with blood. The results of transfusion were miraculous:

I have seen men already like corpses, blanched and collapsed, pulseless and with just perceptible breathing, [who] within two hours of transfusion

[were] sitting up in bed smoking and exchanging jokes before they went to the operating table.

Hayward's praise of the orderlies working in the resuscitation tent was unbounded as this description indicates:

… a wonderful lad, a boy of 20, he had served without relief for months in this tent, attending to the worst cases and the dying. He had all the patience, tenderness and devotion of a woman, the gentle hands and skill of a nurse and an enduring fortitude.

When he awoke refreshed after his first sleep for thirty-six hours, Hayward looked around and saw a cultivated land untouched by war in his location. He described the air being alive with the songs of larks in fields of poppies and marigolds. The camp and country was a picture of peaceful calm and beauty. If only he could have forgotten the scene inside the tents and close by:

That evening we took in nearly 200 Australians who had been caught by gas shells without their masks on … temporarily blinded and in agony with the difficulty of breathing … it was a weird site to see them led away through the camp in the moonlight in long single files, holding onto each other and guarded by an orderly as leader … our casualty clearing station was ordered to take up quarters with two others in a huge deserted asylum close to Amiens in expectation of the grand attack of the Fourth Army around Villers-Bretonneux. On that evening our barrage opened – a continuous roar of heavy guns which shook the ground and trembled the walls of our building and the sky and fields were lit up with the flashes and explosions of dumps and star shells. In the early hours of the morning came the ambulances in a continuous stream.

Batches of 200 injured men at a time were processed and then shunted through adjoining casualty clearing stations for further attention. Stretchers filled every room and flowed out into the corridors which became blocked by the congestion in narrow, sheltered passages. All the while, nine surgeons were operating simultaneously but making little impression on the masses of wounded, many of whom waited hours without help, or died before they got attention.

A quick surgeon might get through fifteen or twenty cases in a spell of twelve hours. I certainly could not do more than ten or twelve. Amongst so many cases it was a sickening thing to have to make a choice for operations. We were dealing with a mass, not individuals and, if selection had to made, it had to be made in favour of those who by operation had a chance of being made fit again … to return to the Front sooner or later to keep up our manpower and afford fresh fodder for the guns.

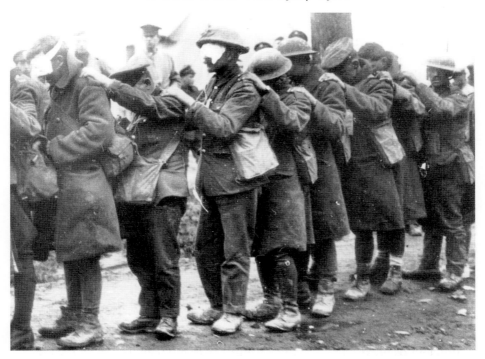

Men blinded by poison gas on the Western Front awaiting treatment. (*R. Ruggenberg*)

In such circumstances nothing seemed to matter. It had to be got through somehow. Action, doing one's best, rightly or wrongly, mistakes or no mistakes, precluded all thought of self and drove out fear and anxiety. All that day and the following day, when the visiting teams began to arrive, we worked. Night shifts took our places and on the following morning I went around the vast building to see what was happening. The wounded, including many Germans, had now overflowed from the rooms and corridors and were lying in stretchers on the open squares of the asylum. Through the night, with dimmed lanterns, doctors and orderlies went down the rows doing what they could, but we were snowed under and we could neither operate on nor evacuate cases fast enough to make much impression on the heaps.

It seemed to Hayward that many of the Germans dreaded they would meet with rough treatment, clasping the hands of the British surgical teams with imploring looks and despairing gestures to convey their fears. They were treated with the same care and given the same priorities as the British injured. On one occasion Hayward came upon an outbuilding strewn with corpses and a pile of freshly amputated arms and legs – the ugly realities of war as he saw them.

It was a week before they had cleared up and evacuated the influx of wounded men, leaving everybody exhausted. Obviously, there was insufficient time for the medical staff to ideally process the number of casualties that could occur in a battle of that magnitude but, as he said:

> It was a famous victory. A lull in the fighting for a few days on our immediate front now ensued and we had some rest. I even went butterfly hunting and on another day went up to the Front and saw our guns firing and heard the German shells coming over and bursting. I remember, one night, we had to spend operating on a number of men, brought in dressed up for theatricals, some of them as girls in ballet costumes. A German aeroplane had dropped a bomb through the tent onto the stage and the tent had collapsed on top of the crowded audience and the dead and wounded.

For Hayward, it was a series of violent contrasts which made up his memories of France. Outside the tents, the sun and the birds and the butterflies and the flowers flourished. Occasionally he was invited to bridge, picnics and concerts. Inside the tents, nature had been violated and outraged. The contrast hardly seemed possible, but it became part of the memory of his first 'blooding' at Crony and Amiens, where he came so near to personal collapse and disaster.

With the advent of long-range artillery bombardments, there was a massive transformation of the conditions of combat. Troops and medical staff were placed under physical and psychological stresses worse than any previously experienced. They fought and worked in massive areas of cratered terrain, added to which was the dehumanising effects of huge battle areas swept by bullets, shells and gas that inhibited all movement. Commanders and troops suffered isolation and disorientation with later campaigns lasting many months longer than earlier battles. Violence on the battlefield reached new and terrifying dimensions and contact between men and medical care became less predictable than ever before. Inevitably, men began to lose hope of ever getting out of their predicament.

In Western Europe, nearly 10 million infantrymen from both sides died as a result of the war. The foot soldier suffered far more than any other military personnel. On the first day on the Somme in July 1916, 20,000 men from Britain and the Commonwealth were killed and twice that number were wounded. No single day of the Second World War compared to the battle of the Somme for the sheer number and rapidity of casualties. Half of the men the surgeons treated had been wounded in earlier fighting and had returned to duty. In fact, it has been estimated that 150,000 of all those injured in the First World War had been wounded more than twice – some as many as four times. Never before had battle surgeons witnessed injuries of such complexity and scale as those inflicted by the large, new shells and shrapnel. Great surgical advances finally occurred from the experience of the war, but that was of no

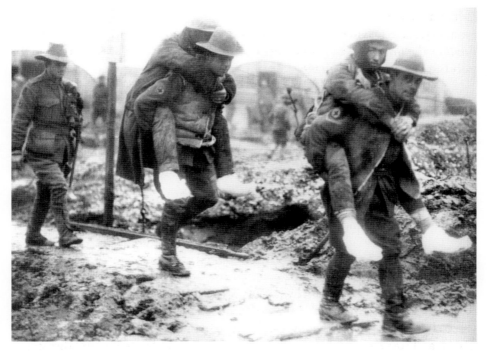

First World War casualties with trench foot being transported by hardy medical personnel, many of them non-combatants. (*R. Ruggenberg*)

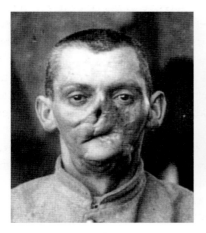 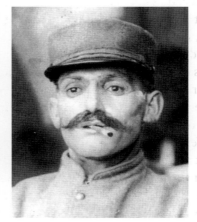

Above left: A Frenchman's blasted face with permanent deformity, First World War. (*R. Ruggenberg*)

Above right: Final reconstruction of the face, employing a left half-face mask for life. (*R. Ruggenberg*)

help to those butchered in the first two years of conflict. Men with serious injuries who survived long enough to be treated far behind the battle lines were finally transported to England, where hundreds of specialists were waiting to put them back together again – for most, that was a step too far.

BEYOND EUROPE

With Germany threatening to bring Turkey and the Moslem nations of Central Asia and North Africa under the banner of the Central Powers, the British and the French took steps towards protecting their bases, colonies and communications in those regions. To that end, British, Australian and New Zealand forces were sent to Egypt to face the Turks. Holding the Turks on the Suez Canal was their first objective, followed by the invasion of Turkey via Gallipoli and the Dardanelles.

After several spectacular battles in which General Edmund Allenby broke the Ottoman Empire's 400-year hold over the area, he triumphantly entered Jerusalem in December 1917. Earn Dole's *Allenby's Military Medicine: Life and Death in World War I Palestine* has recently heaped high praise on Allenby for what Dole regards as his unique success in amalgamating military and medical administrations in Jerusalem during the British occupation.

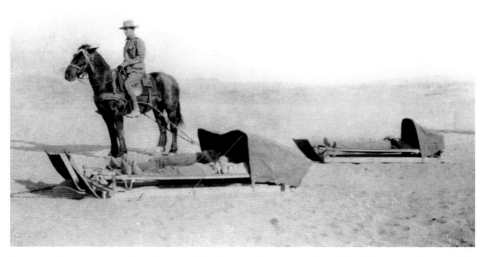

One- and two-man sand sleds towed by horses for evacuation of the injured in the Middle East, First World War. (*Digger History, ANZ Armed Forces*)

Sir Robert Storrs was appointed to govern the city and repeatedly directed Allenby's attention to the need for medical and civil reconstruction programmes, refurbishment of hospitals, vaccinations for rampant diseases such as malaria and smallpox, comprehensive dispensing of medicines and surgical services, and the building and repair of roads and sanitation systems.

AUSTRALIANS AT GALLIPOLI

No country is so wild and difficult [that] men will not make it a theatre of war.

– Ambrose Bierce, American writer, 1842–1914

The Australians and New Zealanders landed at Anzac Cove on 25 April 1915. In their first battle, these same Australians found they had been landed on the wrong beach at the wrong time with little or no support. They suffered terrible casualties in an impossibly rugged and inaccessible terrain, but it was no worse a blunder than that later repeated in the Somme, when they were directed from their trenches to inevitable slaughter.

An official sent by the British War Cabinet to observe the Australians at Gallipoli reported glowingly to his Prime Minister:

I do hope that we shall hear no more of the 'indiscipline' of these extraordinary [Australian] Corps [men] ... I don't believe that for military qualities of every kind, their equal exists. Their physique is wonderful and their intelligence of a high order.

Regardless of the tragedy that followed, tribute must be given to many in the medical and surgical units serving in all areas of the peninsula. Gardner's biography of Captain Henry Wade, a surgeon in the Scottish Horse Mounted Brigade, described the ghastly scene at Gallipoli with its makeshift trenches ripped apart and its bloody battlefields littered with many thousands of dead and wounded British, Australian and New Zealand troops:

In breeches and riding boots, Captain Wade trudged through the misery, tending to the wounded and gently closing the eyes of those for whom his skills as a surgeon were not enough. Wade firmly believed that, "... the surgeon must go to the wounded man and not the wounded man to the surgeon". For that, he equipped an old Wellesley [car] for mobile surgical operations with an operating table, instruments, dressings and a steriliser. Other cars were shipped out to Gallipoli later for the same conversion and variations on his idea have been used by countless armies since then.

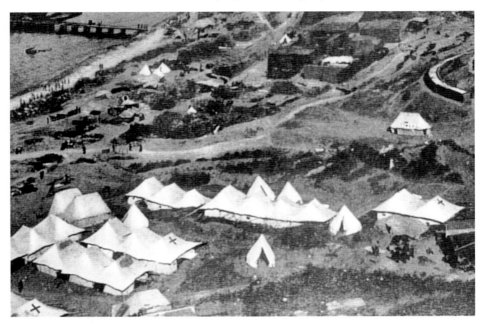

Tent hospital on the shore of Anzac Cove, 1915, overwhelmed by numbers of wounded. (Three Years with the New Zealanders *by C. Weston*)

A member of Wade's team later wrote:

> I had the great good fortune to be one of his [Wade's] assistants on Suvla Bay. Patients brought into the [operating] theatre would say, "Is this Henry Wade's place?" and, when assured that it was, would remark, "Well, if anything can be done to save my life, he is the man to do it." Wade's contribution to field surgery didn't end there. He believed that the important fact in warfare was to do with transport and the sooner a patient was transported to hospital, the better, even if they had to use sand sledges and camel ambulances.

Michael Tyquin, a prominent historian, is one of many who has written extensively of the Australian Army Medical Services in the Dardanelles in 1915. His accounts of that campaign and other events are exhaustive, highly informed and fundamental to understanding what went wrong and why. He exposes the unglamorous reality of that part of the war with its huge casualty numbers, disease and serious medical maladministration on all sides and at all stages of management. He harshly questions the popular images of 'glory, heroism and noble death' and the complimentary stories of military and medical administrations at Gallipoli. In his book, Tyquin includes a 'circular memorandum to medical officers and nurses on hospital ships and ambulance carriers' – confidential advice from Sir Ian Hamilton, Overall Commander of the Mediterranean Expeditionary Force (War Office, 5.12.1915):

All grades and degrees of the medical staff must make it a point of professional honour to maintain a hearty tone of optimism calculated to raise rather than to lower the confidence and courage of the fighting men who have been temporarily committed to their charge ... let medical officers and nurses on hospital ships and ambulance carriers see to it then that, under all trials, they surround their sick and wounded with an atmosphere of enthusiasm and of invincible hope.

Tyquin's 'medical war' refers to the conflict between the medical bureaucracies of Britain and Australia, the poor training of the Australian Army Medical Corps, the lack of political interest, and the inefficiencies and mistakes which led to appalling numbers of casualties. To him, Gallipoli was a makeshift campaign with inadequate preparation. Fortunately, ether and chloroform were freely available and surgical care ultimately improved for the majority of the wounded, but those with head, chest and abdominal injuries rarely survived.

The ambition of all surgical treatment in the field was to move patients as quickly as possible to a hospital ship, even in the face of powerful Turkish opposition, treacherous terrain, bad weather, disorganisation, bureaucratic conflict and a huge surgical load that overwhelmed medical services. To make matters worse, medical help was limited by insufficient personnel, drugs and

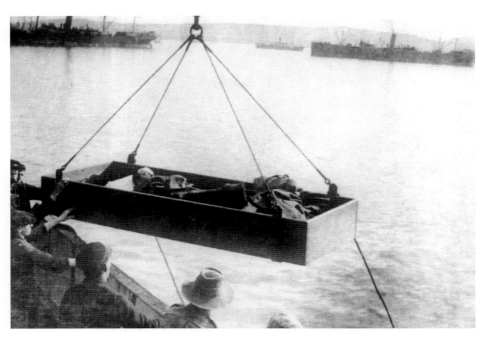

A wounded man being hoisted onto a hospital ship, Gallipoli.
(*Alexander Turnbull Library, New Zealand*)

equipment, and low numbers of small evacuating vessels to feed the hospital ships. One senior commander at Gallipoli revealed:

> ... the outcry, both in Australia and among our own men ... led to a great deal of feeling against the Imperial authorities ... officers say they considered it was murder and would lead them to report to their government that under no conceivable circumstances would they advise the Commonwealth of Australia to enter again upon any war ... under the authority of the British Headquarters, a view that the Australian Colonel John Monash endorsed, "... the British hospitals here – well – the sooner they hang somebody for gross mismanagement, the better."

Tragically, it seems clear that on top of the physical difficulties of the campaign, professional incompetence hindered the delivery of medical services. Everyone recognised that the 'old-boy' network between military services had rapidly collapsed. Relationships between the army and the navy were strained and

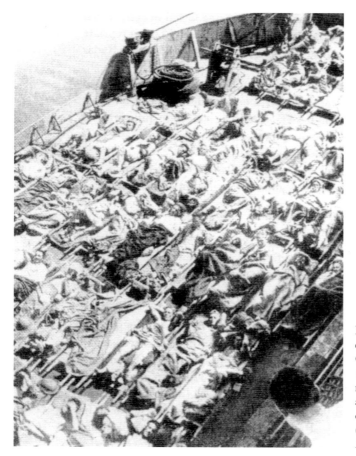

En masse casualty evacuation from Gallipoli beaches, 1915; the sheer numbers precluded adequate processing on hospital ships. (*Alexander Turnbull Library, New Zealand*)

the movement of evacuating craft was poorly managed. Much of the so-called organisation seems to have been frankly incompetent if not negligent.

As they waited for help, medical officers were demoralised and frustrated by their inability to overcome such severe inefficiencies. Behind the scenes, the Australians suffered the same problems as other nations in the Mediterranean Expeditionary Force: self-mutilation, disobedience, shirking, cowardice and dishonesty were affecting the performance of all units to an increasing extent.

Despite his many criticisms, Tyquin's summary of Gallipoli concluded with more favourable observations on later events:

> ... [AIF medics] addressed hideous wounds efficiently, helped intelligently to adjust splints to compound fractures, gave chloroform hundreds of times and assisted at operations. All this was done in a quiet matter-of-fact way, no fainting, no vomiting, just a steady attention to duty ... added to such pressures were the additional occupational hazards of bullets or shrapnel which such personnel shared with all who found themselves on Gallipoli.
>
> The Australian Army Medical Corps at Gallipoli ... [finally came] under the resolute leadership of capable officers ... problems [were] largely resolved by the time the Gallipoli campaign drew to a close.
>
> It was out of the brutal tragedy of Anzac that a tradition of medical care and organisation was born ... the Australian Medical Service came out of the Gallipoli campaign sobered ... [but] ... having served its sick and wounded admirably.

The events at Gallipoli are reflected in the actions of John Simpson Kirkpatrick ('Simpson'), an uncomplicated and forthright man from Newcastle-upon-Tyne who took up mining on the New South Wales south coast in 1910, and enlisted as a stretcher-bearer in 1914. He insisted that he would never fire a shot and apparently never did. It is said that he personally rescued some 300 wounded men at Gallipoli by carrying them on a donkey to the care of surgical units.

Stretcher-bearers had to carry wounded men in full view of the enemy and under fire to makeshift places of first aid, but Simpson used the hardy, agile donkeys that he found grazing among the wounded to transport casualties. He made more than a dozen one-hour trips every day, twice as rapidly but probably less comfortably than conventional two-man stretcher teams, but there is no record of complaints from the wounded.

A fellow stretcher-bearer has left a detailed description of the circumstances of their work:

> Many snipers being in the hills made the carry down the gullies rather unhealthy ... beset with all sorts of inconceivable difficulties ... the carry had to be done without relief over a very muddy and narrow track. At various places ... it was necessary to sprint past these 'warm points' from one place

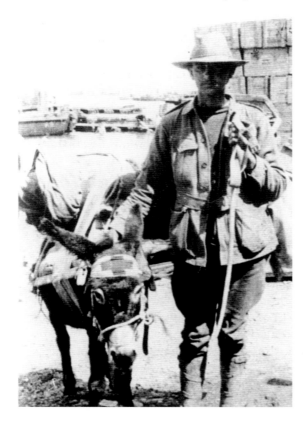

John Simpson, the legendary medic who died at Gallipoli, with his favourite retrieval donkey, 'Duffy'. (Five months at Anzac Cove *by J. L. Beeston*)

to another, and snipers were very diligent and accurate, and shrapnel was also uncomfortably plentiful. Jack used a number of donkeys which he called by a variety of names but his favourite was 'Duffy'. The hard fighting throughout the day caused heavy casualties and the bearers had inadequate means to do their work. The shortage of stretchers was relieved in a measure by improvised equipment sent ashore by the warships, but the need was still so great that it inspired Simpson to commandeer a stray donkey.

One of Simpson's commanders wrote of him:

At the landing on April 25 ... Simpson went ashore with his bearer squad of four. Three of those were either killed or wounded and Simpson was left alone. He only carried men wounded in the leg, [and some with head wounds]; that is, men who could sit astride a donkey with assistance. He left the serious chest and abdominal wounds, those who had to be stretchered to the beach, to the scant resources of the two-man bearer squads available. Colonel Monash fully recognised the value of Jack's self-imposed role, stating that "Simpson was worth a hundred men to me".

Some idea of a battle scene faced by stretcher-bearers can be gained from the following memoir of someone who was actually there on the landing beach:

I don't know what it was, shrapnel, maxim [machine-gun], or rifle fire – I was frightened to look, but I was never so frightened in my life as when I had to stand up [to exit the boat] ... in my imagination I could feel the damned things hitting me all the time, while we couldn't see the other boats from the spouts of spray all around, and the hit men whelped and whined and clawed the air as they died.

At first, the beach was absolutely swept with machine-gun and rifle fire so that there was no possibility of going near the boats or to help the wounded lying on the beach ... three stretcher-bearers were killed and another fourteen were wounded ... then came the awful time ... a man in front of me was shot through the head and a couple of others were wounded ... I felt an awful smack on my side and I knew that I was shot. I crawled for about five yards and found that I could not go any further. So, as the bullets were whistling all around, I put a few stones around my head and laid there for about fifteen minutes. The boys had chased the Turks back again by this time so I crawled to my mates and they fixed me up. The doctor took the bullet out of my wound. By about 5.30 a.m., the Turks had been driven off the cliffs by superior numbers of Aussie soldiers arriving. Soon after dawn, the rifle fire stopped and we were able to look after the wounded – now shrapnel fire only. There were great numbers of wounded whom it took all the morning to attend to and get away.

It was 3.30 a.m. on 19 May 1915, when Simpson began his day as usual by leading his favourite donkey up Shrapnel Valley to have his breakfast and begin work. He had collected a casualty and was coming back down when a signaller called out to warn him of a Turkish machine-gunner:

[Simpson] waved back in acknowledgement ... [a] machine-gun bullet hit him in the back, carrying him forward. He ended up face down in the dirt. After exchanging a few words with others, Jack made a joking remark in his 'put-on' Irish accent, as his colleagues approached. When they heard someone shouting that Simpson had been shot, [they] came running back and found their mate, with his donkey standing next to him. Others soon arrived on the scene. A bullet had entered Jack's back and passed out the front of his stomach, having penetrated a vital organ. We laid him down carefully, put his body in a dugout by the side of the track and carried on with our job. There was great gloom that night when it became known that Simpson had died. We finished our duty at 7 p.m. and all that was left of our section gathered around our old pal and carried him down Hill Spit where we buried him. A clergyman officiated. A simple wooden cross on which was written only the name, 'Jack Simpson', marked his grave.

Australian Commanders at all levels and the surgeons who manned the primitive shelters in which first-aid surgery was often given believed that Simpson deserved a Victoria Cross, but it seems that, in preparing Simpson's citation, a junior officer recommended him under 'the wrong category of heroism'. Regardless of the many high-ranking opinions in his support, all decorations were denied to Simpson on the ground that they 'might set a dangerous precedent'. Nobody knew what that precedent might have been. To them, Simpson was unique.

Perhaps that attitude makes a connection with one intriguing aspect of Gallipoli that has not been much exposed – the censorship of information revealing the horror and shame of much of that campaign. For example, when writer Sydney Loch, who was there, attempted to publish his experiences of Gallipoli, he and his publisher were threatened with prosecution.

AN ARMY'S WILL TO FIGHT

War is an ugly thing, but not the ugliest of things. The decay and degraded state of moral and patriotic feeling which thinks that nothing is worth war, is much worse. A person who has nothing for which he is willing to fight, nothing which is more important than his own personal safety, is a miserable creature and has no chance of being free unless made and kept so by the exertions of better men than himself.

– John Stewart Mill, British philosopher, 1806–1873

Desertion has affected armies throughout the history of war. It represents an 'unplanned depletion' of an army's potency. It is termed 'external' when men go missing and are never found again, or 'internal' when men stay put but lose the will to fight.

It may come as a surprise that medical staff have sometimes been asked to identify violently anti-social individuals who could seek out exceptionally dangerous missions. While some of these men are effective, many of them are unreliable and go missing, with or without the job being done, never to be seen again.

It would be unrealistic to believe that the availability of rapid, expert medical retrieval services could ever persuade soldiers to leave cover and advance in combat without great reservations, but most did so when ordered. After all, every soldier and many non-combatants understood a lot about fear – but a few men seemed to have no fear at all. Some had plenty but conquered it with various degrees of success. Others feared everything constantly, whether or not they were in danger. Most just bottled it up for the sake of their mates and got on with a job that had to be done and hoped, in one way or another, the war would finish one day for all of them. Few of us would believe that a critical point could be reached in any army when a majority of troops might refuse to go on fighting – but, at one time or another, that precise situation threatened all the armies who fought in the First World War. It seemed most likely to happen after long periods of constant engagement or when the total number of casualties had begun to exceed the number of fighting men still available.

One Australian battalion on the Western Front went 'on strike' because they were the constant 'battering ram' in every major attack. They had, despite earlier brave fighting, simply had enough.

Some leaders believed that competent, sympathetic leadership might delay an unwillingness to fight, especially when some troops confidently regarded their officers and surgeons as being in the image of Christ – a powerful provocation to continue in the face of abject fear.

One of the most disturbing events for any military surgeon is the murder of a fellow soldier as a protest of some sort. One form of this crime has been called 'fragging' (throwing a fragmentation grenade) at an officer who was thought to be incompetent, uncaring or shaming their men by their own courage. Other perpetrators believed that they were not adequately valued and were getting even by killing one of the establishment. It was first reported in the Second World War, and in Vietnam there were more than 1,000 cases, but it is certainly a very much older problem than that.

Not surprisingly, some men resented the prolific and undeserved merit awards given to non-combatants who had never been at risk. As a result, they took their anger out on their superiors. On the other hand, many incidents of 'fragging' showed that pure fear could turn admiration and loyalty into resentment, envy and an urgent need for revenge. The causes are often ill-defined – something that the psychiatrists could not identify. On the eve of the battle of the Somme, many men on both sides took an action that they might never have thought possible for anyone in a proud army. They inflicted wounds on themselves to avoid ever having to fight again. One resentful surgeon on the Western Front described them as, '... the shirkers who generate more shirkers'. Self-mutilation sometimes spread to such an extent that large battle plans failed or had to be revised.

Regardless of the risk of severe penalties, including execution (except in the Australian Army), self-inflicted wounds requiring surgical treatment became more common as the First World War progressed. Some surgeons found them almost too distressing to treat. It was estimated that only 5 per cent of all 'accidental' wounds in that war were genuine, but they were an infallible passport from the battlefield to freedom. Worst of all for the medical groups, these men and their wounds proved exceptionally difficult and unrewarding to treat. Whatever was done for them was bound to fail, often from a repetition or exacerbation of self-damage as soon as they left hospital. Whether or not

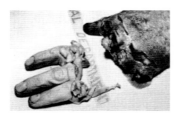

Self-inflicted amputations to evade combat during the
Second World War, as seen in all wars. (*US Army*)

they could properly be called cowards and become candidates for summary
execution, nobody was sure. Many were regarded as operating within the
confines of their normal (for them) but more limited visceral capability. They
were, by any definition, unreliable in combat and the army was generally
considered to be 'better without them'.

The 'esprit' of individuals, armies and nations boils down to whatever produces
'cohesion', a quality that was thoroughly tested in civilians in Britain and
Germany between 1941 and 1945. It mostly seems to depend on a confidence
of adequate and available surgical and medical support if injured. It also relies
on a belief in a good cause, good training, a trust in leadership and, maybe, a
God (sometimes seen in the person of a leader), a sense of honour, good logistics,
decent living conditions between campaigns, pride in a unit, a sense of being
treated fairly and, not altogether surprisingly, an efficient postal service.

Self-inflicted wounds were relatively easy to diagnose, but to include a
doctor on a court martial bench to help determine the motives of an alleged
deserter was an extraordinary demand. He might be asked to determine if the
accused was a true deserter (one who left his post without permission and
had no intention of returning) or an absentee without leave (AWL). Doubts
about the quality of medical care in the event of wounding were important
factors thought to convert some episodes of 'AWL' into 'desertion'. To make
such decisions about either act was often impossible. More than 3,000 British
officers and men were condemned to death for disobedience during the First
World War, but only 350 were executed. For the rest, their sentences were
commuted to terms of imprisonment.

It also seems, despite popular myth, that most soldiers don't fight for a
monarch, flag, cause or country, but rather for their mates – to not let them
down. With troops isolated in battle, 'buddies', 'mateship' and 'peer groups'
may satisfy a 'herd instinct'. The influence of good commanders becomes a
powerful surrogate for the support of family and friends at home. Medical
teams often observed that high levels of personal and group morale and
confidence in their surgeons can greatly delay the onset and number of
psychiatric and even physical injuries. Doctors and padres have peculiarly
similar roles in providing some of those needs.

In many wars up to the modern era, western armies have had a golden rule
that 'no man will be left behind' and, where the situation allows, it seems to be

practised. That alone would be of great comfort to men going into action and contemplating being wounded.

In the early 1800s, Napoleon had recognised that confidence in the availability of high-quality medical care in the event of injury was a major concern of his troops. He combined his own strange charisma and the excellence of his surgical commanders to maintain a remarkable level of morale throughout long campaigns. Behind the scenes, he both dazzled and repelled men by his fluctuations between frenetic activity and laziness, but he openly promoted his best surgeons at every opportunity. Baron Larrey was just such an icon – a 'Saviour' to his men for his energy and courage. Thousands would fight all the harder just for knowing he was somewhere nearby during a campaign.

It is no secret that Anzac troops were considered by many British officers to lack army discipline. After all, one in every hundred of them had been in an army prison at some time and they were often regarded as disobedient, untrustworthy and poor fighters. Others considered them superb fighters. According to Australian War Memorial figures, of 416,800 Australians who enlisted in the First World War, 60,000 were killed and 156,000 were wounded. That was the price paid to persuade the British Army that the Anzacs were a different and worthwhile breed. While Field Marshal Haig's admiration for the Australian soldiers grew, they never ceased to puzzle him when their out-of-battle behaviour conflicted totally with British Army standards.

Senior Australian commander, Lieutenant-General Sir John Monash, was sufficiently incensed by the criticism of his troops that he wrote in his diary:

> Very much and very stupid comment has been made upon the discipline of the Australian soldier. That was because the very conception and purpose of discipline have been misunderstood. It is, after all, only a means to an end, and that end is the power to secure coordinated action among a large number of individuals for the achievement of a definite purpose. It does not mean lip-service, nor obsequious homage to superiors, nor servile observance of forms and customs, nor a suppression of individuality ... the Australian Army is proof that individualism is the best and not the worst foundation upon which to build up collective discipline.

Unlike other Allied armies, Australian soldiers who were arrested for mutiny, desertion or cowardice and sentenced to death were not executed. The Australian government believed that, as volunteers rather than conscripts, these men should not be subjected to the maximum penalty. After all, the vast majority of the Australians who died in the First World War had done so on the River Somme on the Western Front and at Gallipoli where, relative to population, Australia's casualty rate was the highest of all Allied nations involved in the war. Exactly why is not clear, but aggressive AIF attacking techniques may have been one answer, and incompetent generalship another.

CONSCIENTIOUS OBJECTION

Implicit in this concept is 'objection to what?' In the 1960s, an American doctor was charged with refusing to help train Special Forces whose conduct contravened his ethical principles. He relied on his adherence to the Hippocratic Oath as justification for his action, but he was nevertheless dishonourably discharged. His judges included both doctors and military commanders.

There have been many doctors, health workers and others whose religious and ethical positions have dissuaded them from certain military roles or from bearing arms for any reason, but who have been quite willing to serve the wellbeing of the men in hazardous places. Some even engage in activities such as casualty retrieval, parachuting, medical experiments on themselves and, most remarkably, in bomb disposal teams.

A West Point graduate and flight-surgeon who refused duty in the Persian Gulf in the Second World War was fined heavily and sacked from the service, shaming his family by his actions. Why some surgeons agree to full participation in war without being combative and others demand no involvement whatsoever remains a troublesome issue for armies and colleagues to consider. Of course, harsher critics would say that any man who suddenly discovers an aversion to war on the brink of engagement is disingenuous at best and cowardly at worst.

'Simpson of Gallipoli' was a clear example of the sincere objector who would do anything in battle except fight. Cassius Clay was another who claimed a conscientious objection to military service. Many medical opinions were taken about the sincerity of his beliefs – one even venturing that Clay was of subnormal intelligence, a classification that automatically rendered him unfit for service. However humiliated he was by that, he continued to speak out freely and cogently about his beliefs. Nobody could take seriously the view that he was cowardly, of course, but he never fought in war. Thirty years earlier, the Nuremberg war crimes trials established the principle that a fighting soldier must decide for himself which orders are morally unacceptable to him. The judges specifically rejected the defence of criminal conduct on the grounds of obedience to an overriding respect for authority. For the first time known, this new concept ratified the previously theoretical right of a soldier to disobey the orders of his superiors.

CHAPTER 10

Infections, Antiseptics and Antibiotics

Man knew that he could catch an illness from someone or from something – but only vaguely, as he still imagines the chill wind to blow him rheumatics. Even Hippocrates failed to twig onto infection.

– Richard Gordon, *The Alarming History of Medicine*, St Martin Press 1993

'Mother,' complained Achilles at Troy, 'I am terribly afraid ... that flies may defile the corpse of my Lord Patroclus by settling on the open wounds and breeding worms in them.' 'My child,' Thetis comforted him, 'I will arrange to keep away the flies and save him from those pests that devour the bodies of men killed in battle.'

– Homer, *Iliad* XI, 700 BC

In the eighteenth century, when doctors still doubted the value of elementary hygiene, untrained nurses, wives, relatives and cooks, camp-followers were already becoming convinced that diseases such as dysentery, typhoid, malaria, typhus, yellow fever, pneumonia, the common cold, measles, mumps and epidemic influenza could all be reduced simply by isolation and cleanliness. When Florence Nightingale's great influence in the nineteenth century provoked fresh interest in the same beliefs, the stage was set to better educate surgeons, soldiers and commanders alike.

The discoveries of Pasteur, Koch, Lister and others had enlarged the bacteriological knowledge which became accepted by the late nineteenth century. Injecting syringes and needles for drugs became available in 1853. In 1890, an American surgeon, William Halsted, persuaded the Goodyear Rubber Company to manufacture thin rubber gloves to protect the hands of nurses and surgeons from the irritating effects of carbolic acid, which was frequently used as an antiseptic agent in surgical procedures. He soon realised that wearing impervious, sterile gloves also provided an excellent barrier to the transmission of bacteria among those involved in surgical procedures. Ironically, while investigating local anaesthetic agents and post-operative analgesics for military surgeons to use, Halsted and some of his surgical colleagues became addicted to cocaine and morphine. Though still addicted, he continued his surgical and experimental work for twenty-five years before he died from complications of a surgical procedure which he had pioneered.

Definitions overlap between what is an antiseptic and what is an antibiotic. Nowadays, 'antiseptics' are usually regarded as chemicals which can kill germs by being in contact with them, while 'antibiotics' not only kill germs on contact but can also be given by mouth or injection to inhibit their enormous rates of breeding. Antiseptics such as carbolic acid had been pioneered by Lister in the nineteenth century and iodine soon followed. Mercury compounds had been used as antibiotics to treat syphilis but had such awful side-effects that many patients preferred to live with their disease rather than try to cure it. But the hunt for better drugs was becoming urgent. Paul Ehrlich and a Japanese colleague tested the anti-bacterial qualities of nearly a thousand substances in the first decade of the twentieth century, trying to find something that could destroy bacteria from within the blood stream. 'Salvarsan' (called '606' because it was the 606th compound they investigated) was shown to be effective against the germs of syphilis and sleeping sickness, but it was unacceptable because it contained arsenic.

A breakthrough came between the First and Second World Wars when a German biochemist, Gerhard Domagk, discovered the sulphonamide antibiotics for which he was awarded a Nobel Prize. When first used in 1936, they revolutionised the treatment of infections and saved countless lives. Such was their success in treating pneumonia that they were honoured for, 'dethroning the captain of the men of death'. Their remarkable effects were also demonstrated in the French Foreign Legion during an epidemic of meningitis, where the death rate fell from 75 per cent to 11 per cent. They were used extensively during the Second World War, both as a powder to dust into wounds and as swallowed tablets to give systemic and comprehensive treatment. Therefore, within the first half of the twentieth century, there was a dramatic transition from antiseptics, with their limited surface-active capabilities, to the sulphonamide antibiotics with their remarkable ability to inhibit the reproduction of bacteria and destroy them deep within the body.

Viruses didn't concern the surgeon much except for causing 'civilian' diseases in fighting men. Viruses did not respond to antibiotics then as they do now. Bacteria were the germs that caused battleground infections; they rapidly invaded and grew in all open war wounds, particularly those that contained dirt, debris or dead tissue. Without thoroughly removing all dead and foreign matter by physical measures, gangrene was common and antibiotics were largely neutralised.

It was in 1929, the year the Great Depression began in earnest, that something very big happened in the medical world. It changed forever the management of infections in war, civilian surgery and medicine. Alexander Fleming, a Scotsman working at Oxford, noticed one Monday morning that a common laboratory mould, penicillium, had inhibited the growth of

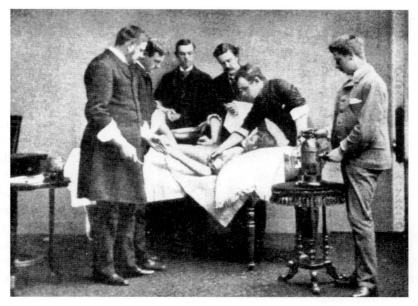

Carbolic spray being delivered from the man on the right to kill germs in the air, with several assistants and Lord Lister about to operate on patient's left arm, apparently without general anaesthetic. (*Richard Gordon*)

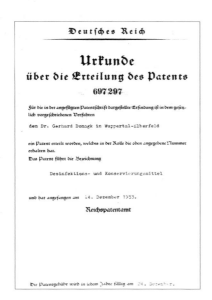

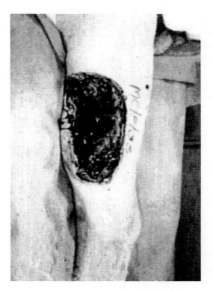

Above left: Gerhard Domagk's sulphonamide patent document, 1933, later printed with a Swastika. (*Richard Gordon*)

Above right: Wide removal of dead tissue from a right thigh wound (no fracture) left open to drain under observation. (*Dr M. Crumplin*)

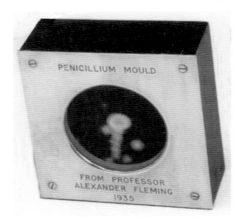
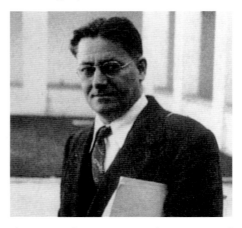

Above left: White spots represent bacterial colonies in Fleming's original experimental dish. The white spots on the dark surface are penicillium mould (from which penicillin is derived) near which no toxic bacteria were growing. (*Richard Gordon*)

Above right: Australia's Howard Florey who redeveloped Fleming's work on penicillin in 1939. (*Richard Gordon*)

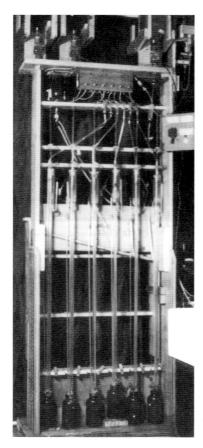

The world's first penicillin factory, filling sterile bottles below from flasks above. (*Richard Gordon*)

staphylococcal bacteria in a culture dish left uncovered over a weekend. He couldn't see then how it could be useful in therapy and put aside his discovery as a curiosity. After all, for centuries the power of various moulds to inhibit infection had been known but not understood.

Ten years later at the start of the Second World War, Howard Florey, an Australian, took fresh notice of Fleming's work. With a pathologist, Roy Wright, and a biochemist, Ernest Chain, he re-studied the way penicillin worked. In 1940, they and their many colleagues were able to show that it was a very powerful antibiotic.

So impressed were they with its potential and so fearful that Britain was about to be overrun by Hitler that Florey's team carried spores of penicillium in the linings of their clothing. They planned that if they were forced to escape a German occupation of Britain, the new wonder-drug might be taken to North America and developed there, solely for the British Empire's use.

Florey visited the United States to get help with the mass production of penicillin and to develop its potential with military surgeons. The enterprising Americans quickly took out international patents on the drug and charged royalties in its war use. It and the sulpha drugs were soon made available to all Allied theatres of war and, before long, to civilians. There is no doubt that penicillin changed the course of history. How many millions have survived wars and civilian illnesses because of it will never be known.

Fleming received great praise for his original discovery of the penicillium mould's effects. Nobel Prizes for Physiology and Medicine in 1945 went to him, Florey and Chain. However, many others had collaborated with Florey in the work leading to the isolation of purified penicillin and its clinical use. It was vastly superior to the sulpha drugs and, if used carefully, carried few serious side effects.

What had never been possible before in the surgical care of serious wounds then became feasible and the rules and nature of battle surgery changed forever. The place of radical, destructive surgery such as amputation to prevent spreading infection could then be considered in a new light. Penicillin was one of the reasons that complicated brain, chest and, particularly, abdominal surgery became possible for the first time, with much better rates of survival than had occurred in the First World War.

CHAPTER 11

Red Gold

God gave men both a penis and a brain but, unfortunately, not enough blood to run both at the same time.

– Robin Williams commenting on the Clinton–Lewinsky affair, 1998

This slick irreverence contains one of the essential mechanisms of the state of 'shock'. When the amount of blood in the circulation fails to match up to all the demands being made on it, some body organs are deprived and may never function again. Major war injuries need blood transfusion if wounded men are to survive long enough to have life-saving surgery.

A normal, average-sized male contains 5–6 litres (10–12 pints) of blood and a female about 4–5 litres. Haemorrhage is the commonest cause of shock in a military setting. 'External' bleeding can be seen and controlled by first aid, but 'internal' bleeding may be difficult to locate if the body's surface is intact.

For example, a fractured shin and severed artery may mean a hidden wastage of more than three pints of blood around the fracture site – rapidly depriving the circulation of a third of its total volume. Worse still, a fractured thigh or pelvis might conceal the loss of more than half of the body's blood content.

Soldiers in the First World War suffered a torrent of bullets and shells that often forced the injured to remain where they had fallen for hours before being collected by stretcher-bearers – if they were lucky. Retrieval was a slow, jolting journey through trenches and open territory to the first level of medical care. Hours or days may have passed before definitive therapy was available; they were often exhausted by the time they arrived at the point of surgical care. By then, without anybody knowing exactly why, many of them were at death's door. In some, blood loss was obvious but other men, with only moderately severe wounds, suddenly collapsed and died without explanation. Before long, for want of a better description of what nobody understood, surgeons said these men were dying from 'shock'. For some reason or another, and even if they hadn't lost much blood, their bodies lacked sufficient quantities to fully fill their blood vessels and maintain their circulation. Toxic substances from wounds could make their blood vessels so 'flabby' that they couldn't maintain a normal blood pressure within them.

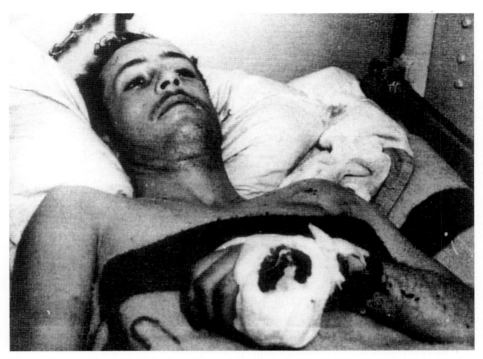

Typical appearance of shock from blood loss after shrapnel wounds to the left arm and hand, awaiting transfusion, Second World War. (*US Army*)

The poor circulation caused by shock means that nutrients are not delivered to body cells, toxic products are not removed and a lethal spiral towards death is imminent. The cold, pale, apprehensive, sweaty patient with low blood pressure is on the verge of irreversible organ failure and death. That was the syndrome that surgeons saw on battlefields and which only a transfusion of blood components could begin to rectify – if it could be done early enough, quickly enough and in adequate quantities.

Blood is pumped by the heart through big arteries into the smallest capillaries at a sufficient pressure to maintain the life of every body organ. About one-half of blood consists of cells – red and white – which have different jobs. Red cells carry oxygen from the lungs to every body cell and then take the carbon dioxide residue back to the lungs for discharge into the air. The pale liquid part of blood, called 'plasma', carries cell food and antibodies as well as white blood cells which fight infection. In blood banks, plasma with the white cells removed is called 'serum'. Depending on the abnormality being treated and what is available to them, doctors can transfuse either 'whole blood' or any one of its components. Whatever is given is beneficial, but whole blood is best of all for the shock state.

Blood transfusion had been attempted from animals to animals and from animals to humans in the seventeenth century. A few experimental animals survived but no humans did and, apart from a few sporadic 'experiments', the procedure was put aside for 250 years. Transfusion had become a symbol of futility.

In 1905, George Crile, an American surgeon (who had previously helped develop the rubber surgical glove) had mastered the clotting and 'compatibility problem' and decided it was time to try transfusion again. He stitched a compatible donor's artery directly onto a hole in the vein of a shocked patient and was able to directly transfuse the sick patient. By avoiding exposure of the donor's blood to air and foreign surfaces, it didn't clot.

Many military surgeons remained resolutely unconvinced of the value and safety of blood transfusion and insisted on transfusing salt solutions only. They preferred to transfer moribund and shocked soldiers to a quiet ward where they were drugged and allowed to die from a completely unknown cause.

Ten years later, the bloody Battle of the Somme showed British surgeons that something much better was needed for wounded men. Surgeons repeatedly observed shock that was far more severe than any of them had ever seen in peace-time practice. The availability and storage of blood were problems they still could not overcome – within a few minutes of putting blood into tube or a bottle, it clotted. Faced with that challenge, a small group of surgeons on the Western Front, independently of each other, had been contemplating a very controversial procedure. Edward Archibald and two other surgeons recognised that blood treated with sodium citrate (a substance related to citrus juice) would neither clot quickly nor harm the patient. The magic of citrate was that it made blood 'storable' for considerable periods without clotting.

Compatibility was already understood following Karl Landsteiner's pioneering work on blood groups. Blood donated by volunteers or convalescent patients could be typed, kept in bottles containing citrate solution and stored at low temperature in a blood bank, or even transported over large distances. At reasonable leisure, it could be transfused into shocked patients; the more blood given, the more rapidly men recovered – to a degree that major surgery was feasible and safe.

Previously sceptical surgeons suddenly recognised the miracle of blood transfusion and that revolutionary lesson was never forgotten. Today's blood banks collect whole blood into bags containing an anti-coagulant solution called 'CPD' – Citrate Potassium Dextrose. The principle is the same as Archibald and others observed nearly 100 years ago. It can be stored in a refrigerator at 4–6°C to avoid the growth of bacteria and it has a shelf life of about three weeks.

For use in remote locations, plasma can also be used to expand blood volume and is universally compatible. Better still, after being harvested from volunteers, it can be frozen, dried and stored in plastic bags for weeks or months. By 1941, the American Red Cross Blood Bank had developed programmes to provide large quantities of plasma for use in the European and Pacific areas – much of

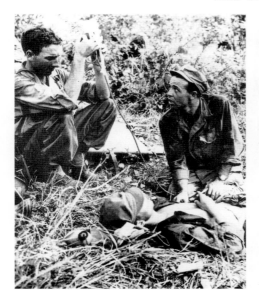 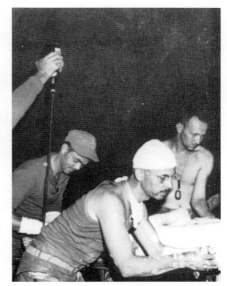

Above left: Second World War medics giving immediate plasma transfusion in the field. (*US Army*)

Above right: Second World War medics transfusing blood in a tent hospital. (*US Army*)

it delivered by parachute – where it saved countless thousands of lives. One estimate was that, for every American casualty in Europe, an average of two pints of blood was given for initial and urgent resuscitation.

By the end of the Second World War, nearly 15 million bottles of blood had been converted into plasma for easy transportation and prolonged storage. General Dwight Eisenhower, Supreme Commander of the Allied Expeditionary Forces in Europe, commented that, 'If I could reach all Americans, there is one thing I would like to do – thank them for plasma and whole blood. It has been a tremendous thing.' At war's end, almost 1½ million units of plasma were taken from army stores and returned to American civilian hospitals. Without the discovery that blood could be stored with the treatment of sodium citrate, none of that would have been possible.

CHAPTER 12

The Second World War,
1939–1945

If a wounded soldier was still alive when the medic found him, he had an
excellent chance of survival ... [The medic was taught to do] ... whatever was
necessary to stabilise the wounded man ... stop the bleeding, lessen the pain,
bandage the wound and get him to the aid station.

– Anonymous war medic, US National Archives, 2000

In terms of numbers of individuals involved and casualty rates, the military historian John Keegan described the Second World War as '... the largest single event in human history'. However, as in other conflicts, its conduct was often affected by the common difficulty in rapid transportation from battle fronts. Wounded men knew that evacuation-crews, medics, ambulances, expert surgery and anaesthesia were often distant from them. Most Second World War casualties never expected the rapid air-evacuation and high survival rates that became common in later wars.

Since Vietnam, fifteen years after the Second World War, retrieval helicopters have become one of the greatest 'surgical implements' available to modern warfare. They can bring casualties and surgical teams together in less than an hour. With compact battle zones and efficient communication, helicopters may land in the open under fire to collect and give first aid to wounded men within minutes of injury – faster than a civilian traffic victim might wait for an ambulance today. It is now an unlucky soldier who dies before receiving treatment for his wounds, but in the Second World War it was a very different story.

The Industrial Revolution of the eighteenth and nineteenth centuries led to sophisticated weapons of destruction and, by the dawn of the twentieth century, military ground vehicles and war planes were already realities. With modern civilisation firmly based on technology, there was then an environment as dangerous as anything nature could ever have contrived. The machine-guns and artillery of 1914 delivered such destruction that men could find shelter nowhere but deep within the earth itself. At any one time during the Second World War there were nearly 50 million men and women serving or being prepared for service in armed forces somewhere. Counting both sides, by the end of the war, over 50 million soldiers and civilians (more than half being civilians) had died – more than seven times the population of Australia at that time. Surgical advances during the conflict were enormous but slow to become universal because of the size of battle zones, the multiplicity of campaigns, the difficulties in dissemination of information and the inadequate numbers of senior surgical personnel who were required urgently in huge and increasing numbers.

Among the Allies, urgent calls went out to hundreds of distinguished surgeons, anaesthetists, dentists, veterinarians, ophthalmologists and psychiatrists seeking their enlistment in the services. On both sides of the Atlantic, army medical departments intensified their educational programmes. Medical schools in America were filled as never before with junior surgeons rapidly training at the hands of dwindling numbers of experienced teachers. After Pearl Harbor, increased collaboration with other Allied forces produced the largest surgical machine of all time, but it had to be spread rapidly across multiple campaigns in widely separated areas.

Compared with earlier wars, the Second World War was fought in vastly different environments that affected both troops and medical teams. The special features of various combat zones influenced the nature of injuries and their treatment. A combat medic, Albert Gentile, wrote a frank and moving memoir of how first aid worked for him in Europe:

> There wasn't a moment when I wasn't scared, but that's a disadvantage an aid man has to live with. He can either control it or demand to be relieved of [his] duties. The thing I discovered in combat was [that] the vast amount of soldiers conquer that fear while there are others who are too stupid to understand the meaning of fear, and they are the most dangerous because they drive to win medals and return a hero ... they take risks that end up getting someone else killed.

Gentile saw no difference between being killed in the Second World War, the First World War or the American Civil War, but the Second World War soldier had chances of survival that were far greater than any of his ancestors. Around 50 per cent of those admitted to hospitals in the American Civil War died. In the First World War, the figure was 8 per cent and less again in the Second World War. Antibiotics like the sulphonamides and penicillin had become available and more advanced surgical techniques were introduced, but the main reasons for improved survival were the speed with which men were retrieved from battle, their urgent surgery and the wider use of adequate amounts of blood transfusion.

> It began in the front line ... medics had been mildly despised because some of them were conscientious objectors and often ridiculed ... the main objective was to get the wounded away from the front lines ... this involved the medic

climbing out of his foxhole and into No Man's Land to collect a fallen comrade. He would ... evaluate him ... inject a vial of morphine, clean up the wound ... followed by a bandage ... [and] drag or carry the patient out of harm's way. At an Aid Station one to three miles behind the line, the [doctor] would remove the bandages, administer blood plasma if needed and [the boy] is rushed back to a point known as the Clearing Company Station far in the rear, carried by a comfortable ambulance.

One of a field hospital's principal functions was to care for injuries of the head, chest, abdomen and thighs that needed great surgical expertise if men were to survive. For that, the general aim was to bring major surgery as close to the front line as possible.

What were later known as 'MASH units' in the Korean War revolutionised early surgical care. They allowed the less-threatened casualties to be transferred quickly to evacuation and field hospitals where skilled, specialist care was available.

A remarkable example of military and medical improvisation was evident in the evacuation of defeated British and French forces from Dunkirk and other Channel areas during nine days of early 1940 – two weeks after Winston Churchill had become Prime Minister. He and Field Marshal Lord Gort had enthusiastic and competent medical support in the expectation of many casualties. A vast contingent of vessels of all sizes and types went from England to collect some 350,000 men (100,000 of them French) from the open beaches of Dunkirk while under fierce German air attack. More than 200 small vessels never returned to England.

According to Gort, medical services were stretched far beyond their limits, but they all coped valiantly. British surgeons provided support not only on the Channel beaches and in small ships, but also in scores of receiving hospitals in England.

TEAM EVENTS

Nothing can diminish the recognition by many that the 'medic' or 'paramedic' is the backbone of modern medical military services. They form the first link of a chain that joins wounding to the possibility of survival. Their contribution makes it possible for surgeons to accomplish whatever good they do.

Nursing is another occupation that has multiple definitions. Their job varies somewhat from place to place and time to time, not only because of the experience of a nurse, but also because of the demands of various locations. Based on the traditions of Florence Nightingale in the Crimea, the ideal roles of battle nurses had become clearly established by the end of the American Civil War and continued through to the Second World War. Just as some doctors cannot possibly confront the prospect of operating on the sick, injured and dying, or even touching them comfortably with respect and sympathy, others can and do so every day. So it is with good nurses who, by instinct, can comfort the frightened and the hurt. Everyday and in every war, they do just that – often in danger in the field, in operating rooms, wards and ambulances. They are the link between surgeons and the sick – between peace and anguish.

Many nurses from many countries volunteered for military duties in the First and Second World Wars – giving anaesthetics, dressing wounds, setting simple fractures, applying first aid, managing artificial lung-ventilation, intensive care, simple dentistry and psychiatry. As a tribute to them, in 1949 the British Royal Army Nursing Corps gained, for the first time, formal military ranks for its members, irrespective of sex and colour.

The US Army Nursing Corps had been established in 1775 during the American War of Independence. By the start of the Second World War in 1939, nearly 30,000 nurses had enrolled with the American Red Cross Nursing Service and made themselves available for overseas service. Within a year, 170,000 nurses had actually been enlisted and there were similar trends in Britain and other Allied countries.

There is an argument that female nurses contribute something different and perhaps more elemental than their male colleagues, probably as a function of their charm and the romantic perceptions of their patients. Field Marshal Bernard Montgomery was one who firmly believed that female nurses had a unique effect on military morale. In his view, no male could nurse the wounded exactly like a woman – a view that is probably shared by most surgeons, patients and male carers. But there is no doubt that all sorts of medics, male nurses, stretcher-bearers, retrieval crews, orderlies and technicians are equally crucial components of medical teams. Their valiant performance matches that of female nurses in everything but the manifestations of that priceless 'X' chromosome of their female gender.

During the Second World War, 60,000 American nurses served near the front lines – 20,000 of them in Europe – with many decorated for exceptional bravery. They were often under fire in the field and in evacuation hospitals, on hospital trains and ships, and as flight nurses on medical transport planes. Nearly 500,000 soldiers were treated primarily by nurses for psychiatric disorders. Nurses taken prisoner by the Japanese were treated no better than the troops whom they nursed. One, who was stationed in a vulnerable location in the Philippines during the Pacific War, recorded the nervous strain of working in the combat area:

> The air ... was thick with the smell of disinfectant and anaesthetics and there were too many people. Several times the power plant was hit, leaving

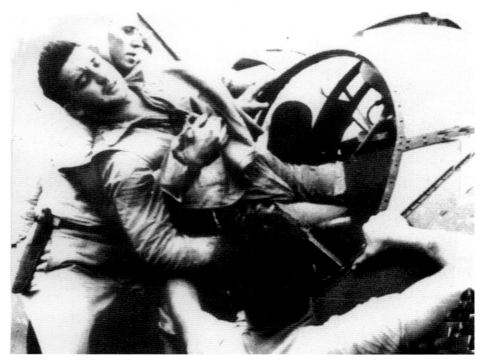

A wounded gunner is eased from his turret after an injury sustained by anti-aircraft gunfire, South Pacific. (*US Army*)

us without electricity or lights [for surgery]. It was pretty ghastly in there, feeling the shock of each detonation and never knowing when we would be in total darkness.

Due to a continuing segregation policy in the first two years of the war, only a small number of black nurses served in the US Army. Later, they were allowed to treat black troops in black wards, but by 1944 public and military opinion and need had forced the reversal of all such discrimination. Many nurses of both colours were wounded when Germans bombed hospital ships indiscriminately in the Mediterranean, just as the Japanese did later in the Pacific. By the end of the war, all military nurses could be commissioned and receive full retirement benefits, dependants' allowances and pay equal to that of men.

One celebrated example of the military nurse's prowess occurred on a heavily laden transport plane that ran dry of fuel over the ocean while en route to Guadalcanal. It carried twenty-four passengers but no doctor and only one flight nurse. When the pilots had to crash-land on a coral atoll, one patient suffered a catastrophic neck injury, which threatened to paralyse and choke him. With no immediate advice or precedent, the nurse improvised a system of

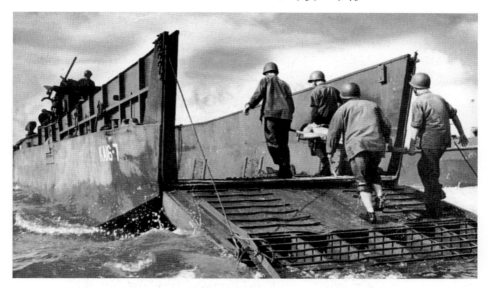

A patient is carried aboard an American landing craft, Second World War, Pacific area. (*US Army*)

splints, tubing and valves from basic articles on board the aeroplane, saving the soldier's life.

It is a tribute to air-evacuation nurses that only a tiny proportion of the 1¼ million patients carried throughout the war died en route. However, seventeen flight nurses lost their lives, some from a flagrant disregard for Red Cross establishments, both on shore and at sea, by German forces.

By 1944, 5,000 American nurses were serving in the South West Pacific and, inevitably, surgeons delegated responsibility to them for many tasks. In the Mariana Islands, they treated men with severe shock from haemorrhage, multiple wounds and traumatic amputations. Those on ships were in constant danger from kamikaze attacks. Looking back on the Pacific carnage, one senior nurse wrote, 'Sometimes I think maybe it's a good thing their mothers can't see them when they die.'

James K. Sunshine is now eighty-four and lives in Ohio where he is an Oberlin College librarian, archivist and whatever else he chooses to be for his old college. He joined the US Army in the Second World War as a private and emerged three years later as a staff sergeant-technician (non-commissioned officer) of the Medical Corps attached to 42 Field Hospital. That distinguished unit was on Utah Beach, Normandy, during the invasion of Europe in June 1944. Sunshine typifies the gallant men and women who worked alongside surgeons and nurses in a myriad of tasks that demanded exceptional courage and devotion to duty. Without such collaboration, no surgeon could operate well and many badly injured soldiers would not survive and no army could fight effectively.

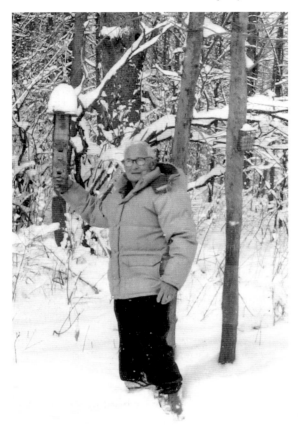

James K. Sunshine, Normandy
medic, in Ohio, Christmas 2008.
(*J. K. Sunshine*)

Other 'medics' similarly engaged were under intense bombardment during
and after Normandy. Some 2,000 of them died during the European campaign
although they wore red crosses on their uniforms and equipment and carried
no arms. Alongside surgeons, nurses, ambulance staff and technicians, they
gave sulphonamides, penicillin and transfusions, and ensured quick treatment
and evacuation of injured troops. They observed the same principles of 'staged
wound management' as had been established in 'MASH' units worldwide.

Sunshine supervised the establishment and operation of his hospital's
surgical programme and assisted surgeons during operations within the
demountable tents. The hospital had 100 beds, 60-odd enlisted men, several
physicians, 6 nurses for tent wards as well as teams of surgeons, anaesthetists
and enlisted men who assisted at operations.

As he describes it now, the procedure was to set up the tent hospital, treat
serious injuries of the head, chest, abdomen and thighs and then move the
hospital on to another location every few days – repeating the performance
at each stop to keep up with the advance as it moved forward. Serious post-

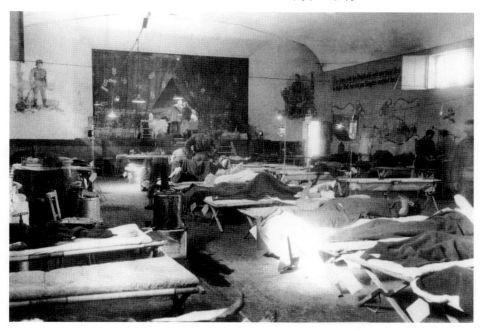

Second World War casualty dressing station (probably German) in a concert hall, with the operating area on the stage with patients treated and waiting. (*R. Ruggenberg*)

operative patients were left in ward tents to be cared for by holding-companies of medical attendants for up to ten days before more formal evacuation.

Sunshine's work provided an unusual vantage point from which to observe the war. He described his job of assisting surgeons:

> … I am told to hold a leg while the surgeon saws it off. I wonder why I don't throw up. The landscape of France is littered with half-destroyed tanks and trucks, blasted houses, dead cows, bodies turning black in the summer sun, stench everywhere. Wounded men, tagged for identification, are lying on litters in rows all over the field. Walking wounded stand around waiting to be helped. Ambulances arrive with fresh loads. Most are American paratroopers … but some are Germans and others are simply unidentifiable foreigners pressed into service by the Germans. The enemy soldiers have been at war a long time and they stink of dirt and sweat and blood. They are given the same treatment as Allied casualties. I dig my hole beside a hedgerow and report to a tent surgery. I am a surgical technician … who works in a surgery and assists surgeons. A surgeon, a major, notices me standing uncertainly and says, 'Let's go, Corporal, get some blood on your hands.' Not really funny, perhaps, but then we all were drunk with excitement and determined to do well. I follow him through the blackout curtain into the surgery where three surgical teams are at work. Generators outside the tent provide power for lights.

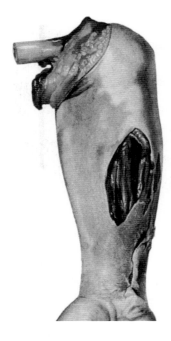

Amputated right forearm to stop the spreading of
gas-gangrene infection from a contaminated wound.
(*Dr M. Crumplin*)

He discovers a German dying in an isolation tent, but taking a long time about
it; there is the smell of gas gangrene; neither can speak the other's language.
The young, blond, filthy man cannot survive but the surgeons amputate his legs
and he is hurried away as far as possible from the other wounded lest he infect
them. The operating tent and instruments and everything the man has been in
contact with must be sterilised urgently before they can be used again:

> The night sky is lit by flashes of artillery fire ... a few yards away, the steadily
> growing hospital dump smells of burning, bloody bandages and discarded
> flesh and limbs ... with the exception of an occasional undertaker's assistant,
> none of the technicians has had previous medical experience [in war].
> Building on the experience of World War 1, the army has decided to move
> major surgery as close as possible to the most seriously wounded, operating
> on them immediately, while less seriously wounded are moved back to
> evacuation hospitals in the rear. Most seriously wounded, means men shot
> through the head, lungs, bowels or large bones of the legs, wounds that in
> World War 1 were usually fatal.
>
> Our basic technique is to open up a man's abdomen with an eight-inch
> incision, go through the intestines and other organs carefully, looking for
> holes made by bullets or shell fragments. Damaged organs and bowel are
> removed, the holes sewed up and the incision closed excepting for a loop
> of bowel which serves as a temporary outlet. Minor wounds are cleaned
> of damaged flesh and packed with Vaseline gauze. We do chests as well as

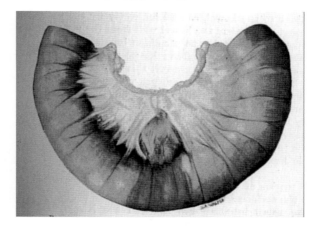

A removed loop of bowel showing destroyed blood vessels at 6 o'clock, allowing leakage and severe infection. (*Dr M. Crumplin*)

bellies, sometimes on the same man. We use great quantities of whole blood. We have sulpha which we smear liberally everywhere we can and everyone who lives gets the new drug, penicillin, every four hours.

The surgery tent is big enough for two operations to occur at once on men lying on their litters supported on saw-horses. Each patient has two surgeons, an anaesthetist and a surgical scrub technician. Another technician stands by to replenish instruments and do odd jobs that the surgeon needs. Every couple of hours, they move on to another patient.

It is a quiet night. Sixty men fresh out of surgery are sleeping on canvas army cots. I go from cot to cot with a syringe loaded with penicillin, thrusting it quickly into each man's buttock ... most of them are too sick to care. I check IV fluids and suction, give water, take temperatures and try to ignore the subdued moans of pain that have become a steady background ... men who have lost arms and legs are the worst. Some of them, I think, simply talk themselves to death. And most nights, two or three men in each tent die and their bodies are placed in a truck that waits outside. Each morning it makes the trip to where digging crews bury them in temporary cemeteries. Once, we placed a French woman in the truck, thinking she was dead. She wakes up and there is hell to pay.

We become expert at our medical jobs and efficient at setting up the hospital in two hours and taking it down a few days or a week later. The landscape around is littered with half-destroyed tanks and trucks, blasted houses, dead cows and, in the hedgerows and woods, German and American bodies turning black and bloated in the summer sun. We keep moving. Without knowing why, we are told to change shoulder patches from the 1st Army to the 3rd Army and are given over to the newly arrived General George S. Patton whose idea of war consists of speed, violence and 'always wear your helmet, soldier'.

Nearly half a million Allied troops were wounded in Europe. Those who could be treated had an immediate mortality rate of about 5 per cent. The more seriously wounded were sent on for reconstructive treatment by specialists in more than 100 major military hospitals in Britain, some with a receiving capacity of 750 to 1,000 beds.

As the Battle of the Bulge began in December 1944, Sunshine's group was located in a three-storey house, pock-marked by shellfire. The Germans had broken through the Ardennes forest for one last offensive drive. In retreat, his group had to leave behind non-transportable patients with a surgeon and technicians who volunteered to stay. He discovered later that they were soon captured by the Germans, but treated reasonably. On Christmas Eve 1944, he saw hundreds of American aircraft filling the sky.

Sunshine's most admired surgeon, Lamar Soutter, was a chest specialist who had volunteered to be landed, with others, by glider near a town where there were a thousand casualties lying in a warehouse.[1] They were under the care of a single surgeon who had no blood or plasma. Nine surgeons and technicians with fresh blood and drugs were landed in a snow field at the edge of the town and, on the first day of their assignment, the team completed fifty-six operations.

One morning in 1945, sleeping in a battered house being used as a hospital, Sunshine was woken with the words, 'Wake up! Roosevelt is dead. Truman is President and it's time for your shift.' He had never heard of Truman. He went into the surgery to relieve another technician. 'I am told to give a patient on the table a pint of plasma. My hand shakes so much I cannot find the vein.'

As the European war finally wound down, Sunshine recalled, 'Our trucks roll through the devastated rubble ... villages whose streets are lined with cheering crowds, who throw bottles of Calvados and fresh vegetables into our hands ...' His group came across a camp run by the Germans, full of starving men and heaps of corpses. At Buchenwald they found more piles of corpses alongside naked, skeletal men lying on their wooden bunks in tiny cubicles. No civilians in the area admitted to knowing anything of what had happened in the camp. The German troops he saw in Munich in May 1945 were mostly old men and fourteen-year-old boys, some barely able to carry a rifle. There he also saw a scene out of 'Dante's Inferno' – crowds filling the streets as they looted the bombed-out remains of buildings and shops. A man in concentration camp garb comes out of a cellar with a two-gallon jar of dill-pickles and he

---

1. In certain areas of the European campaign, gliders played a critical role for both sides in the evacuation of the wounded and in the delivery of troops, medical teams, guns, vehicles, tanks and blood, often in advance of the fighting. Their value lay in their silence and ability to 'land' men in particular areas with greater accuracy than by parachute. Inevitably, most were sacrificed after use.

and Sunshine party on them and fine Rhine wine. In the morning, a constant stream of newly liberated Allied soldiers and German prisoners were walking aimlessly down the highway – Americans, British, Indians and French – and they share chickens, pickles and the remains of the wine. The war was just about over in Europe.

After the European war, Sunshine returned to Oberlin College to finish the studies he had left when he enlisted in early 1943. He later gained a master's degree in journalism from Columbia University in New York and worked in senior editorial posts for nearly fifty years. On his eightieth birthday in 2004, he recounted some of his remarkable memories to me:

> I had the good fortune to be a surgeon's assistant in a forward Field Hospital, back from the line just far enough to avoid getting shot, but close enough to feel I was part of a huge war machine that could never be defeated. Although it was not my doing, I seemed fated to be on the edge of many of the great moments of that part of the war. I watched the sixteen-inch shells from the battleships fly over my head onto Utah Beach, trying to bring down the church steeple shielding German gunners. I assisted surgeons cutting off arms and legs and digging shrapnel out of the bowels of wounded GIs. I put up and put down the tents of the 42nd Field Hospital sometimes twice in the same day, moving it forward to keep up with the line of battle from St Mere Eglise to east of Munich.
>
> That summer I lived with bodies, American and German, rotting in the hedgerows, and dead cows rotting in the fields. That winter I escaped from St Vith in the Bulge one step ahead of the oncoming German infantry I could see on the hillside. I rode in a fleeing truck convoy past Malmudy two hours before Jochen Peiper's SS group massacred their American prisoners in the snow-covered field. I was at Buchenwald the day it was opened up, gagging at the sight of the emaciated prisoners and horrified at the sight of piles of guards who had been beaten to death by the inmates.
>
> I remember it as if it were yesterday, the thrill of sailing aboard a troop ship into New York Harbor, past the Statue of Liberty, to see the huge sign: "Welcome Home – Well Done". It was May, 1945 and the Pacific War had yet to be won. I nearly cried.

AMERICAN MILITARY NURSES

By the end of the Second World War, more than 200 American military nurses had died, some from enemy fire – six of them were killed in Italy in 1944 by deliberate German bombing of a hospital. In 1942, more than 100 US military nurses were captured by the Japanese in the Pacific and remained in concentration camps for more than three years. Nearly 2,000 nurses received combat decorations of all grades. A supreme Allied commander referred to them as 'those good soldiers' and in the words of one of them:

> [We] ... had to assume a lot of responsibility ... as there were not enough doctors to supervise every case at every stage ... endless harrowing hours ... giving injections, anaesthetising, ripping off clothes, stitching gaping wounds, of amputations ... comforting the wounded we could not save ... seeing people torn and bleeding and dying.

Nurses in a POW camp in the western Pacific told how an American doctor had begged the Japanese for medical supplies to treat sick prisoners. The Japanese finally agreed and escorted him to a truck to collect them. There were two shots and he was never seen again.

As they were demobilised, a small flood of highly trained nurses in specialties such as anaesthesia, psychiatry, administration, teaching and the organisation of evacuation hospitals found themselves back on the US mainland. Many of them became involved in these capacities in civilian life and they and others have done so with distinction ever since. Their elevated status has remained a benchmark for nursing standards worldwide.

The famous British writer, Lucilla Andrews, worked as a nurse in June 1944, when 150 flying bombs were launched onto London daily. From St Thomas's Hospital, she looked down on the Thames to watch the bombed city, wondering if the destruction would ever cease. On one especially bad day, five operating tables were working simultaneously and non-stop in her hospital to shorten the queue of casualties arriving for urgent treatment.

She witnessed the results of the evacuation at Dunkirk – malingerers and hypochondriacs mixing among the gravely wounded. She arrived at work one morning to find a great queue of ambulances:

> Rows and rows of stretchers, loaded with men lying so still that at first we thought they were all dead. They were all covered with grey blankets and their faces were dreadful ... greying-black and sort of slimy, but caked ... men had their eyes open and could move their lips so we knew they weren't dead but they didn't look living.

She later nursed Australians of the AIF and wondered about them:

> [Did they know] ... how their fathers had talked and laughed before the Dardanelles and if as many of the sons, as the fathers, would die before reaching home again ... I had come to realise war was a killing business and that those most likely to be killed in war were the young men in uniform ... long-jawed AIF faces that even on the slightly older men looked ... touchingly

youthful ... so far from home ... in a strange country ... as disturbing as the thought was, still apparently totally ignoring the cost to themselves.

AUSTRALASIAN SURGEONS

If there is anything better than one pint of blood, it is two pints of blood.

– Australian surgical motto, 1944

The accounts written by many gallant Australasian surgeons surpass many others for their detailed and practical observations of the conditions in which they worked. Although miraculous results were often attributed to the availability of sulphonamides and penicillin in New Guinea in 1944, there were many sceptics. All agreed that thorough wound cleaning had a great influence on healing and had to be done at the first encounter.

Wounds had to be scrutinised daily to ensure there was no deep infection and that clean healing was occurring but, by the very nature of battle, there was interruption of observation while a soldier was being evacuated. The rule was that a history had to be attached to every patient with written notes, particularly on plasters, splints or dressings, to tell the next carer exactly what had been done, why, when and by whom.

Surgeons soon discovered how to deal with almost any problem on the spot and in the worst conditions – with none of the refinements of civilian hospitals back home. Different groups found similar ingenious solutions to difficulties in widely separated areas, with no prior collaboration or teaching. Obviously, British rules of 'best practice' surgery were universally known and applied by Australasian surgeons who, in those days, had all done their senior surgical training in Britain.

One senior Australian surgeon was severely deaf. If nearby gunfire or bombing was loud enough to distract his attention, he would remove his hearing aids, knowing that his assistants would know exactly what he wanted, just from his habits and gestures. 'Those buggers were absolute mind-readers ... we never let each other down, not once ... we got on like a house on fire ... once or twice that was exactly where we found ourselves when we were bombed.'

Surgeons in North Africa were relieved to find that 'the desert was kind' when it came to infection. It was said that no patient in Libya or Syria had gas gangrene on arrival at a casualty clearing station although 90 per cent of wounds involved limbs below elbow or knee and many were open fractures with deep contamination.

The dry, supposedly sterile dust of the desert infiltrated huts at a rate worse than that of the Australian out back. To minimise the physical soiling of instruments and wounds, and for aesthetic and practical reasons, surgery was often performed in a small tent pitched inside a larger tent. Surgeons wore gloves, masks and Mackintosh aprons because sterilised linen and gowns were in short supply. All agreed that early closure of major wounds was almost a criminal procedure, regardless of the 'sterile' atmosphere of North Africa. There was always another day on which to act or regret what was done, but the safest approach, if only for observation, was to leave all wounds open in the first place.

At that time, it was regarded as a blessing to have anaesthesia by an injection of Pentothal followed by ether gas. The combination gave soldiers instant, dreamless sleep – a great mercy and safety for those whose wounds required immediate, intensive debridement and other treatment in forward areas, and for those men who required rapid evacuation and definitive surgery elsewhere.

Early in the Second World War, the harsh, age-old pragmatic principles of triage in battle surgery were reiterated for Australian surgeons by B. Rank and H. Poate:

Many battle casualties are still potential fighting men and it is essential that maximum functional results are obtained in minimum time. Where possible, the primary requirement is to maintain troops at their full fighting strength. With that subject in view, it is essential to give preference to the battle casualties who can be returned to duty within a reasonable time. Of course, surgeons' sympathies would always go out to gravely wounded men, such as those with abdominal wounds (which carry a 50 per cent mortality) and the total unfitness for service of another 50 per cent who do recover. Such cases had to be subordinated to those who could be returned to their units within a short time.

This reorientation, this change of mental attitude, by which the preservation of the soldier as a fighting unit assumes prime importance, is not always easily obtained ... without sacrifice of the qualities that go to make a faithful surgeon ... he might have to jettison much of the technical details and proprieties of civil surgery. Resource, quickness in decision, speed of execution and ability to being able to stand the stress of long periods of concentrated work are called for and are indispensable to the successful practice of war surgery.

One of many unattributed reports of the Libyan campaign of 1941 described the appalling conditions of a major dressing station:

... In four days, almost 1,300 men, sick and wounded from New Zealand, British and South African forces, plus German and Italian prisoners were brought in for treatment. Considerable numbers of German wounded were being admitted [also, and the colonel] arranged for the release of two German medical officers and a number of medical orderlies from the prison-of-war cage to assist with the treatment of their own casualties. The German officers … proved pleasant and cooperative in every way. An attempt was made to pass the Italian wounded to the German medical offices for treatment but they politely sent them back. The New Zealanders found that the German medical orderlies avoided all contact with the Italians.

The reception centre was frequently choked with waiting cases, stretchers with wounded covering the entire floor of the large tarpaulin shelter, with many more outside men with gaping, horrible wounds and piteously smashed and broken bodies, but there was hardly a murmur from them. Their courage and endurance were amazing. Blood transfusions could be given only sparingly but wounds were dressed and fractures splinted. Day and night in the theatre, with the thick smell of blood, ether and antiseptic in the air, work continued. The nursing orderlies could not hope to give these men the care they really required. Food had to be strictly rationed and water was so scarce that Red Cross invalid foods could not be prepared for the serious cases.

Joe Koefod, who died in Pottsville, New South Wales, in 2007 at the age of ninety-four, spent three and a half years as a gunner in the Australian 7th and 9th Divisions in North Africa. He recalled that malaria and dysentery were rife. Shell-shock was common but, after a rest period and some ineffective form of counselling and medication, most sufferers were rapidly returned to duty despite their continuing anxiety.

Joe suffered his own agony when a 'friendly' artillery shell exploded within yards of him as it was being loaded into a gun. After first aid and a few weeks of rest, he returned to normal duty, almost totally deaf. The blast had damaged his hearing forever and he certainly experienced manifestations of shell-shock, such as violent nightmares and anxiety for the rest of his very productive civilian life. He once told me that the best survival advice he ever had was from a battle-experienced American platoon sergeant, Burt Evans, in 1944. According to his widow, Joe still recalled the advice sixty years later:

The first mistake recruits make under fire is that they freeze and bunch up. They drop to the ground and just lie there; won't even fire back. I had one man just lie there while a German came right up and shot him. He still wouldn't fire back. When a machine-gun opens up, the new men squat right where they are. The same when flares drop and bombs [come] down at night. The old man doesn't stay out where he is exposed. He dives for cover. When you hear a sharp crack over your head like popcorn, or just like a bullet going through a target on the rifle range, that's the time to duck. Don't worry about the sniper who hits around your legs. The guy to fear is the one who puts a shot close to your ear – 'ping'! He has telescopic sights.

2/4 AUSTRALIAN GENERAL HOSPITAL (AGH)

Dr Rupert Goodman, eminent in the field of education, served as a nursing orderly with 2/4 AGH in the Middle East, Indian Ocean and South Pacific. He has recorded that it dealt with nearly 15,000 casualties at Tobruk and 10,000 in Jerusalem, Colombo and Labuan. Some hospital staff were shipwrecked off the North African coast and others were killed by bombing. Nine members of Goodman's unit died while serving – three of them doctors and four of them medics.

A foreword to Goodman's book contributed by Major W. B. James, who later lost a leg in Korean combat but still became a distinguished surgeon, includes an 'insider's' comments about primary care:

> For a young healthy man to be suddenly incapable of caring for himself, to have to rely on others for the most intimate of care, is perhaps as great a shock as is the medical shock of the injuries. I vividly recall my gratitude for the devoted care of the medical and nursing staff ... and particularly their empathy in my moments of anguish. Their work, then, was but an example of the very ethic of the care of the sick and wounded in war.

In 1939, there were an estimated 13,000 trained nurses living in Australia, of whom only 600 were in the militia. When called on, there was a flood of volunteers who, if they were to satisfy the stringent requirements of the army, needed to be:

> Trained, doubly registered, experienced, British subjects living in Australia, single, between 25 and 35 years of age for overseas service and below 40 for matrons, passed A1 medically and of good character with personal attributes essential to the making of an efficient army nurse.

2/4 AUSTRALIAN GENERAL HOSPITAL IN TOBRUK

We had never encountered such defensive tactics, nor faced such a determined opponent [as the Australian troops] ... [British artillery] and the discipline of the Australian infantry had defeated the German blitzkrieg tactics. [You] are extraordinarily tough fighters. Once [our] tanks got through in Poland, France and Belgium, the [enemy] soldiers took it for granted that they were beaten. But you are like demons. The tanks break through and your infantry still keep fighting.

– German battalion commander, Tobruk

… immensely big and powerful [Australian] men who, without question, represented an elite formation of the British Empire, a fact that was also evident in battle.

– Lieutenant-General Erwin Rommel, North Africa

A regimental medical officer, who wishes to remain anonymous, confirmed to me the accuracy of the following description of the situation existing during the Siege of Tobruk:

[we] … were receiving wounded direct from the 'front-line' with a dressing as the only attempt of treatment. This meant that we functioned as a combined Field Ambulance, Casualty Clearing Station (CCS) and General Hospital … the work in the theatre … was bloody in every sense of the word. Owing to the withdrawal of the [nursing] sisters, the work fell upon about half a dozen orderlies who were totally unprepared for the tremendous responsibility.

[There were] … two tables in two small rooms and to these the wounded were brought in as they had been picked up, in filthy, blood-stained clothes. Their clothes were cut off them. Some were operated upon without this even being done … In these theatres during rush periods, only gut and head wounds were operated on. The main ward [had] eight sets of trestles built to take a stretcher at a convenient height for operating. To each two sets there was a small anaesthetic table and stool, and a wheeled trolley for instruments.

They had soon developed a procedure for the arrival of the big convoys of wounded: patients who were quickly examined and brought down to the operating area to be lifted onto a stretcher placed on a trestle. An orderly cleaned the man's skin as the anaesthetist began his job. Another orderly brought a trolley up to the table and the surgery began with an ample supply of instruments such as would be used in any modern operating room in a civilian hospital. The orderly who had cleaned the patient's skin with antiseptic, then scrubbed up and assisted the surgeon during the operation.

… when the MO finished one case it was only a matter of scrubbing up and moving straight on to the next because the orderly who had assisted him would wheel the dirty instrument trolley out to the sterilising room … and then reset the trolley for the next operation. By … having a team of bearers to bring in the patients and remove them, we did, I think, 90 odd cases in eight hours. The sisters, no doubt, would have gone grey overnight at some of the blunders that were made, but … it wasn't long before all these chaps could do a good job. Of course our asepsis wasn't 100 per cent because we worked without gowns and gloves, but all other precautions were observed. The uniform for operating seemed to be shorts, boots and rubber apron; one surgeon wore his tin hat.

Goodman observed many men in the besieged Tobruk who were labelled with a diagnosis of 'war neurosis' – yet another term for 'shell-shock'. They were breaking down under the strain of months of bombing and strafing that struck both medical and military targets. Some said the worst sufferers had neurotic families or a past mental history. Others were considered unsuitable for further military service simply because they had mental and physical exhaustion after fighting in the desert for the first time. Some were openly fearful of capture and others felt they were increasingly expendable as the siege continued. A few doubted the capability of their medical teams, but there is no evidence to support that view when statistics show that, throughout the siege, 500 surgical operations were performed monthly.

One unsympathetic psychiatrist summed up men with anxiety states as being, 'fed up, blown up, signed up and having the wind up'. Another medical officer concluded reasonably that, 'The main cause of war neurosis is fear. The anxiety and terror inevitable in modern warfare is the exciting cause of almost every case of war neurosis.'

In Tobruk, shell-shock was rarely documented in doctors themselves or their teams, but there is anecdotal evidence that it did occur. The medical staff had a higher level of physical protection than many soldiers and they also worked within an integrated team in a rewarding occupation. While they didn't have to confront the enemy daily as their patients did, they were often in great danger behind the front.

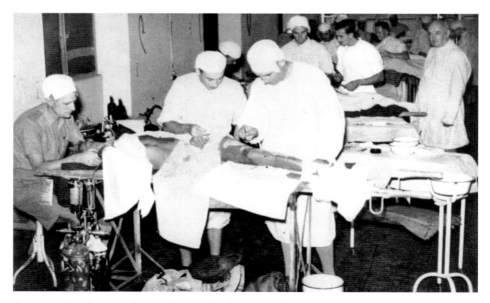

An operating theatre of 2/4 AGH in Tobruk, 1941; there are two operating tables, with the anaesthetist to the left. (*Dr R. Hoy*)

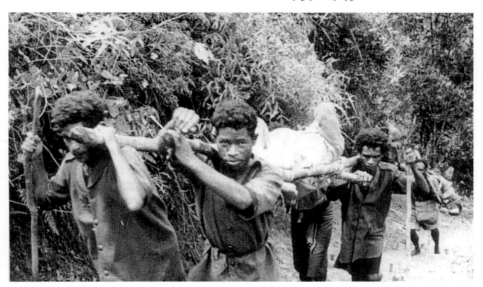

Evacuating the wounded by native labour on the Kokoda Track (or Trail), New Guinea, Second World War. (*Unknown origin*)

Despite great hardships, the hospital's official war diary recorded that, in a six-month period during 1941, the 600-bed hospital in Tobruk examined nearly 35,000 personnel, admitted nearly 15,000, evacuated 8,000, operated on 3,000 and lost only 234 patients from various causes.

With Japan's attack on Pearl Harbor on 7 December 1941 and its rapid advance through southern Asia and the South Pacific, the AGH, together with most Australian forces, was returned home where it prepared to cope with a direct Japanese assault from the north and to receive casualties that would arise from that. After July 1942, they were handling casualties from the frightful conditions of the Kokoda Trail in Papua, a campaign that was being recognised as one of the most heroic and successful defensive actions in military history. Not only were there heavy combat injuries and losses, but typhus had become a serious killer. These casualties were later managed by 2/4 AGH on home ground.

On 5 August 1945, there were 400 patients in 2/4 AGH in Queensland when news came of the atomic bombing of Hiroshima and Nagasaki. Everyone realised that the end of the war was imminent. A short time later, released prisoners of the Japanese (of all nationalities) were also sent south to be treated by the hospital. Many of them were found to have experienced remarkable Japanese brutality and were suffering from extreme malnutrition and uncontrolled tropical diseases.

SURGEONS' DIFFICULTIES IN THE SOUTH-WEST PACIFIC

Don't do any operating. Conditions will not allow it. Your job is to see that the wounded are travelling alright.

– Senior advice to a newly arrived surgeon, Buna, 1942

The evacuation of wounded proved a hazardous undertaking and on this account it was decided ... that operations would be performed as far forward as possible. It was regarded as absolutely essential that we should receive our casualties within eight to twelve hours. The arrival of practically all the wounded at night, and the necessity of very strict blackout made the work more difficult. The unit was situated in a sago palm swamp and water used by the unit was obtained by digging with a spade to a depth of twelve inches. As the battle progressed, supplies became scarce and towards the end of the battle, conditions became really primitive.

– J. M. Yeates, Surgeon, Buna, 1943

The Kokoda–Gona–Buna–Sanananda campaigns accounted for 2,000 dead and 4,000 wounded Australians. The Kokoda campaign alone caused nearly 700 Australian deaths; many more were wounded and even more put out of action by non-combat illnesses that were categorised as 'diseases'.

Half the wounds were complicated open-fractures caused by grenades, shells or mortars. Compounding the problems of infection were heavy rain, lack of aircraft and flooded airfields which delayed air evacuation to Moresby for days on end. Inevitably, established infection or gangrene affected almost all wounds of troops arriving for specialised treatment in Port Moresby at that time. An occasional man needed repair of deep wounds to head or shoulders from Samurai swords.

Where they were possible, front-line surgical operations were routinely performed under tents or tarpaulin covers on operating tables constructed from bush timber and ammunition cases. Surgical tools were sterilised by boiling in biscuit tins on primus stoves. Long lines of natives brought stretcher after stretcher of badly wounded patients through rain storms day and night. Most of them arrived in the late afternoon so that the heaviest surgical demands occurred at night when battery-operated headlamps proved invaluable to surgical teams.

A recurring issue in all locations concerned the number of hours that surgical teams could or should work without rest. If there were no realistic limits, after a few days without sleep for the teams, operating would cease completely. In the interests of productivity, there were frequently two or three operating tables working simultaneously in the same tent with their instruments pooled on a large, central table.

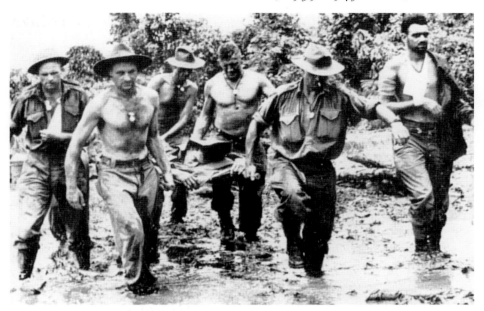

Hot and wet conditions in the Pacific Islands made transport difficult and encouraged infections from contaminated soil. (*US Army*)

In a single day, it was possible to process eighty casualties, but it was generally agreed that the day's surgery should cease after eighteen hours, simply because there were no back-up teams. Of course, that meant that some patients had to wait for hours while the surgeons slept, but there appeared to be no alternative if the work was to continue. Choices were made easier when realistic triage had clearly showed that any unconscious soldier with a severe head wound and most of those with significant abdominal wounds would die whatever was done for them.

Dr James M. Yeates, having calculated that six was the minimum number of hours of sleep he needed to function safely, would give orders that he was not to be disturbed on any account during his rest. He trained his medical orderlies to be competent enough to give transfusions and routine first aid without supervision while he rested. On awakening, he would find a fresh batch of patients ready for their operations. In one frantic period, he and his team performed ninety-eight operations in two weeks. During another period he operated on eleven patients with abdominal wounds – the majority of whom survived – seven limb amputations and ten deep wounds of the buttocks.

Yeates frequently reminded his staff of a comment from the First World War:

For a doctor fresh from a palatial, well-ordered hospital, who has hitherto had all things made easy in view of his training and surroundings, and who may be so confident of obtaining good results that he dreams of performing

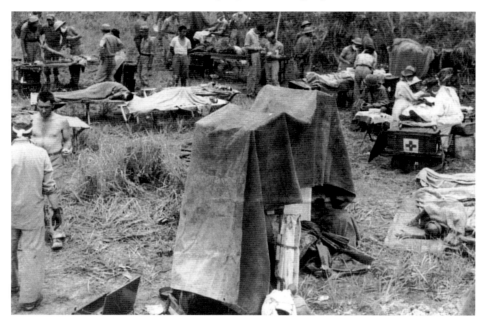

Improvised outdoor shelter for patients awaiting surgery, Burma, Second World War. (*US Army*)

marvellous operations at the front, there will be much to learn and much to unlearn. The dimly lit dugout dressing station, the dust, the wet, the mud, the blood, the noise, the bustle, the numbers of wounded, the appalling wounds, the hopeless shock ... will open his eyes, test his capacity and resources and tend to break his heart as never before.

AIR FORCE INJURIES

Air power is an unusually seductive form of military strength because, like modern courtship, it appears to offer the pleasures of gratification without the burdens of commitment.

– Eliot A. Cohen, 1994

Air crews have unique and intrinsic medical problems by the very nature of being isolated in cramped quarters within their aircraft, exposed to high speed, cold and high altitude, with a proximity to explosive materials such as fuel. Dangers include explosive hits by missiles, burns, cold injury from inadequate cabin warming and trauma from ejection or bailing out. Cold injury at altitude is similar to the frostbite and trench foot of ground troops but without prolonged moisture.

The magnitude of losses and the vulnerability of air crews were demonstrated in June 1943, when the US Eighth Air Force in Europe lost 147 out of 376 bombers during one particular raid. In each of the lost aircraft, there were five or six highly trained airmen and none survived. A major task for medical officers was to help maintain morale in flying groups when the risks of mission-flying were frequently extreme.

The British Bomber Command lost over 47,000 aircrew in action while the RAAF 460 Squadron, which flew raids over Germany, had one of the highest death rates with over 970 KIA.

For medical personnel in the Second World War, the advent of aerial bombing meant much larger numbers and areas of ground casualties, both military and civilian, with wounds similar to those of intense artillery bombardment. It quickly became apparent that surgical teams would have to cope with repeated, indiscriminate, widespread, high density civilian and military casualties. On top of this, there were the special problems of surviving air crews who often suffered burns, blast and cold injury, and compound wounds from shrapnel.

Understandably, in warm climates air crews chose to remove as many of their garments as safely possible in combat – gloves, goggles and even helmets – in order to facilitate their cockpit movements or keep cool. Inevitably, burns from ignited fuel affected heads, necks, chests, eyes and hands. Many of them were otherwise physically intact while all were highly trained and hard to replace.

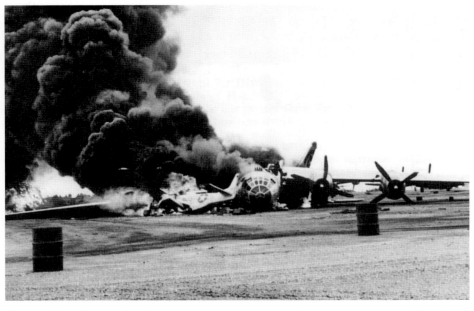

The crash landing of a bomber carried an extreme risk of burns, fractures, crushing, facial injuries and death, Second World War, South Pacific. (*US Army*)

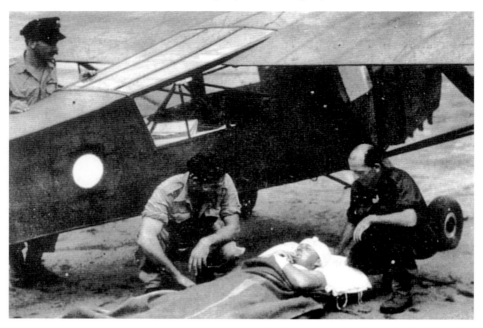

A head injury patient ready for emergency evacuation in a light plane before deterioration can occur, Second World War, Pacific. (*US Army*)

A patient with extensive mutilation, typical of a crash landing, required major, staged reconstruction, including tracheotomy, to enable him to breathe. Expert plastic surgery became an urgent surgical requirement for the multiple stages of 'plastic repair' of disfigured and disabled air crew. Archibald MacIndoe, a New Zealander and pupil of Harold Gillies, earned everlasting praise, and a knighthood, for his pioneering work in reconstructing the faces and limbs of airmen and others in England during the Second World War.

Since the Second World War, refinements of fixed-wing aircraft and helicopters have led to the development of unmanned stealth aircraft, precision-guided weapons and cruise missiles that limit the number of aircrew members. Modern, remotely-controlled 'drones' are crewless – no doubt such military developments and sophisticated weaponry have brought new medical challenges. At the same time, the development of instrumentation for night-flying helicopters and of pressurised, fixed-wing aircraft has enabled critically injured ground troops to be evacuated rapidly, even if they need to be carried at high altitude to places of surgical expertise.

Peculiar to air force wounds from shells, a condition noted in Europe and again in the South West Pacific in the Second World War, was the infiltration of tiny aluminium fragments into exposed areas, so small they could not possibly be removed by formal surgery. No harm resulted apart from disfigurement, but it left a characteristic frosted-glass appearance on X-rays. So long as the

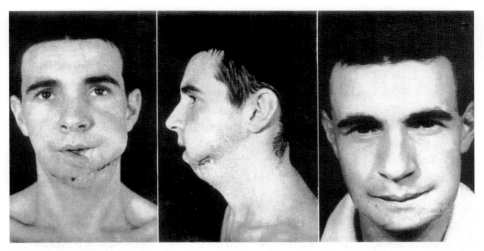

Gross facial injuries repaired in stages to allow a return to civilian life. (*US Army*)

'peppering' was cosmetically acceptable, the fragments were often left in place. Ideally, those that were visible were debrided by 'brush-scrubbing' under anaesthesia as other injuries were being treated.

NAVAL WARFARE INJURIES

War at sea also brought different medical problems. At one naval hospital, sixty cases were encountered in which large metallic fragments from a shell fired from about 20 miles away were lodged inside men's brains. None of them was removed immediately due to the usual difficulty in getting immediate, expert neurosurgical expertise and the unknown prognosis of leaving such foreign bodies where they were. After transfer to specialised neurosurgical facilities for observation, only two of the sixty cases developed a brain infection that required surgery, presumably because most fragments were sterilised by the heat of their delivery.

Lieutenant-Commander John Jeppesen of the Royal Australian Navy (RAN) has described how most, if not all, of the practices of the RAN in the Second World War were based on longstanding British precepts. In 1798, the Royal Navy (RN) had decreed that 'no sick are to be kept below the upper deck of any line of battleship and that a sick-berth is to be prepared in each ship under the forecastle on the starboard side with a round house [latrine] enclosed for the use of the sick'.

Having large fleets, heavy combat demands and an increasing number of wounds caused by long-range cannon, the RN came to regard sick-berth attendants, either male or female, as the backbone of their health services.

On all ships, however, the majority of their patients had diseases unrelated to combat. Since the earliest days of the naval health service, exclusive naval hospitals had nurses who were often the untrained widows of sailors and marines. The medical officer in charge was required to satisfy himself that his nurses had 'moral character, bodily health, strength, sobriety, humane disposition and general fitness'. It was left to Florence Nightingale to introduce even higher standards of nursing in the Crimea where old sailors, often disabled from war wounds and senility, were called 'sick attendants' while the term 'nurses' was reserved for women. By 1884, sick-berth staff, commanded by surgeons, required much more stringent preparation and expertise, each with a duty to '... attend exclusively on the sick, without being called away by the ordinary duties of the ship, and to be paid as an able seaman'.

Based on such patterns, the RAN Medical Service was established in 1911 with fifteen permanent medical officers and a reserve of others in time of war. Dr Alexander Caw was the first doctor appointed to the service and proved to be an extremely competent surgeon under all sorts of difficulties, often operating at sea on patients who needed to be lashed onto tables that were fixed to the floor of the sick bay. The Australians had learned practices such as this very rapidly, which is reflected in the notes of Fleet Surgeon Derby on board HMAS *Sydney* in its celebrated action with the German raider *Emden* off Cocos Island in 1914:

The *Emden*'s guns soon hit us and within five to ten minutes the first wounded man was brought below to me by members of an unengaged gun

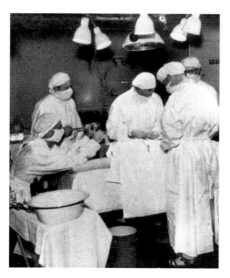 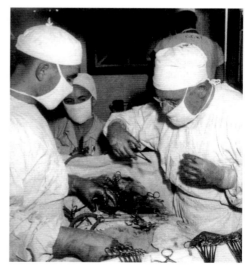

Above left: Operation for appendicitis on HMS *Kenya* at sea. (*US National and Navy Archives*)

Above right: Repairing bowel injuries on a US cruiser at sea.

crew ... most of the wounded were got below by manhandling which was quicker and less awkward. A constant stream of wounded men required urgent attention. The strain had been tremendous and [one of the seamen and I] needed a drink of brandy to keep going. Our clothes were saturated with blood and perspiration and, altogether, it had been a terrific two hours of high tension. The wardroom now contained eleven cases and most of them were restless and groaning in agony. During the action, the space below seemed like a mad inferno. The room was full of men belonging to the ammunition and fire parties and, at the best of times, there was little room here, so the constant supply of wounded men was considerably hindered. We could hear the shouts for ammunition and the continued rapid fire of our guns overhead.

The wardroom was rigged as a hospital and lotions, dressings and instruments were placed handy. The extent of their injuries could not be [determined] until the cases were under anaesthetic. One rescued German sailor had been in the shark-infested sea for nine hours. Another was badly wounded in the leg and abdomen. It was impossible [due to shortage of space] to do any operative surgery until the following day. Early next morning, we arrived off Cocos Island before steaming back to the beached *Emden*. We now had the sick bay rigged up as a theatre, having shifted the beds to make space. The shortage of trained operating theatre staff caused much delay in preparation of each case and the actual operations.

Later in the day we organised theatre staff from volunteers [whose] composure was astonishing since they were present at many bloody operations engaged upon some awful sights to which some of them had not been previously accustomed. Surgeon Todd acted as anaesthetist and [another doctor] assisted me with the operations. One German surgeon on *Emden* had been unable to do much and for a short time was a nervous wreck, having had 24 hours attending, single-handed, so many wounded on a battered and beached ship, with none of his staff left and very few dressings, lotions and appliances. The state of things on board *Emden* was described as "bloody awful". Many were lying killed and mutilated in heaps of large blackened flesh wounds. One man had a horizontal section of the head taken off exposing mangled brain. The ship was riddled with gaping holes and it was only with difficulty that one could walk about the deck. Some of the men who were brought off *Emden* to HMAS *Sydney* presented horrible sights and, by this time, the wounds were practically all foul and stinking and maggots a quarter of an inch long were crawling over them. That is only 24 to 30 hours after injury.

[About 40] of the cases were serious, the rest being more or less slightly wounded and these were able to help themselves ... the condition of many was pitiful; some had legs shattered and just hanging on and others had shattered forearms. Others were burned from head to foot, others had large pieces of flesh torn out of limbs and body ... several were stone deaf [from blast]. The worst sight was the poor fellow who had his face literally blown away, his right eye, nose and most of both cheeks were missing, his mouth and lips were unrecognisable, the tongue, pharynx and nasal cavities were exposed, part of his lower jaw was left and the soft tissues were severed from the neck ... I had no hesitation in giving [him] a large dose of morphine immediately, cleaning the wound as well as possible and applying a large dressing, before removing him to the fresh air on deck. The patient lingered for some six hours [and was given] ... repeated liberal doses of morphine.

The stretcher parties were kept very busy ... sorting out cases to send off next day to *Empress of Russia*, an armed liner which had been despatched to help us with the wounded and to relieve us of some extra 230 men. Fortunately the weather was calm and about 60 patients and 100 prisoners were moved in two hours. A fresh supply of blankets was obtained from the Russian ship as most of those belonging to HMAS *Sydney* were thrown overboard as they were most horribly filthy, foul and offensive and we had no chance of disinfecting them for a long time. Between then and Saturday night we had every case thoroughly overhauled and we were able to discharge

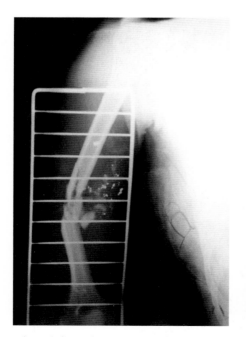 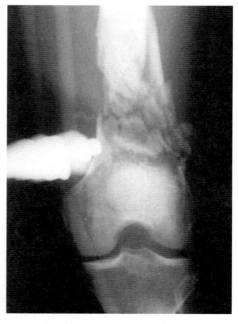

Above left: A shattered upper arm (humerus), splinted and awaiting surgery to immobilise the fracture site. (*Dr G. Peoples*)

Above right: Shattered right thigh just above the knee by a massive IED metal fragment. (*Dr G. Peoples*)

them on Monday in a fairly clean condition, although most of them were septic.

By this time, the ship was in a filthy condition and stinking in all parts near the wounded from their foul wounds. We arrived in Colombo [two days later] where military authorities took over the wounded in military [and civil] hospitals. It would be difficult to imagine a more trying set of circumstances for the medical staff of a cruiser and an action where so many wounded would be rescued. Had the *Emden* sunk before she reached the beach, our work would have been halved as many wounded men [would have] drowned.

During the Second World War, the nursing staff of RAN ships were essentially controlled by the army although some volunteer nurses were appointed directly to the navy. Many of them served in New Guinea and a few were on sea duty. For administrative reasons that are difficult to understand, apart from a hint of male preference in the early history of the British Royal Navy, the RAN Nursing Service was abolished in 1948 and replaced by the Women's Royal Australian Naval Service (WRANS) in 1952. It has served with distinction in Vietnam, Cambodia, the Persian Gulf and Iraq.

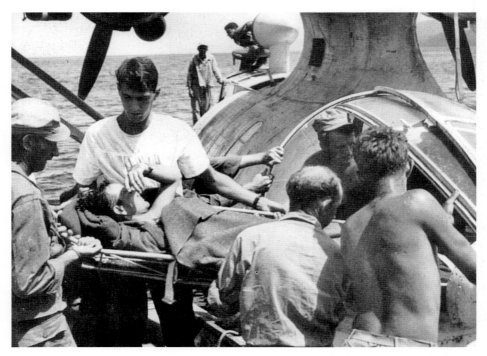

Evacuating the wounded by small airplane, New Guinea, Second World War. (*US Army*)

THE SECOND WORLD WAR:
EUROPE AND NORTH AFRICA

The point is this: we all want to protect ourselves. We have to conserve manpower. We have to stop [soldiers] getting out of the army [if they] can do any kind of a job at all. Can we ever be in a position to say that there is nothing wrong with this man? He might walk right out and drop dead. That is just too bad. We have done everything we can, but it is going to save hundreds of other people for duty if we establish a policy and stick to it ... we have to get out of the family doctor's psychology here and we have to know that we are going to make some mistakes. Can we keep those mistakes down within reason and can we prevent a lot of mistakes being made? If we can almost break 50/50 on it, I think it will be worth trying because we have to conserve manpower.

– US Chief Surgeon P. A. Hawley, 1944

Surgical consultants, who advised army surgeons but did not personally operate, had been invaluable elements of Allied surgical teams in the First World War. When Japanese aircraft attacked Pearl Harbor on 7 December 1941, the Americans entered the Second World War and their Surgeon General suddenly had to confront many crucial issues, one of which was, '... what was the role to be played by consultants in a brand new war involving all combat areas?' It was soon decided that, above all else, they were responsible for the '... maintenance of efficient and smooth functioning' medical teams – no doubt a difficult assignment. Their role was easy to state but hard to make work. Just as the British had found, they had to be relevant to campaigns in Europe, North Africa and the Mediterranean and in the most widespread areas of the Pacific.

There were many components to be considered, the most serious and immediate of which was to shuffle through lists of active army surgeons and those who might be enlisted and sort them all according to their capabilities. Despite the urgencies of the sudden involvement in the war, that task took time to determine and their ultimately ideal deployment had to await the demonstration of their clinical talents in battle areas.

At first there was obvious friction between consultants and senior active army surgeons who resented another tier of command. It was soon clear that the consultants would attend to the things that operating surgeons had no time to do – and probably didn't want to do. Those tasks included keeping records, correspondence, writing reports, evaluating surgical talent, training and the overall integration of surgical activities into widespread areas of combat.

Particular contributions came from senior US consultants, Colonel (later

Brigadier-General) Elliott C. Cutler, recruited from the Harvard Medical School and Peter Bent Brigham Hospital, and Colonel Ashley W. Oughterson from the New York Hospital and Cornell Medical School. They provided meticulous documentation of events and difficulties encountered in their posts and showed how they dealt with them. Some of their despatches beg tantalising philosophical questions about all modern warfare: why do surgeons and their teams choose to go to war, or to terminate their service? What is the dollar-cost of killing a soldier? Is amputation too easy a solution to major limb injuries? Is it acceptable to allow medical treatment to produce a suspension of death to leave a race of individuals with minds and bodies scarred beyond all reasonable recovery? Can medical staff be directed to modify their attitudes to such issues? Does guerrilla warfare impose an impossible logistic challenge for effective medical servicing?

In 1944, the official duties of American consultant surgeons and those of other nationalities were generally defined as follows:

> ... to observe [but not undertake] the care of patients; to ensure the availability of medical facilities and equipment; to determine the professional capabilities of medical officers and their best deployment; to maintain ethical and therapeutic standards; to promote leadership and morale; to keeping proper records and to supervise educational matters.

Essentially, surgical consultants had to assist with all the organisational needs of the clinically active surgeons. The hardest part for the consultant was that he had to supervise surgery while foregoing the satisfactions of performing it, even if he was or believed he was the best surgeon in the army. He was the primary factor in controlling the standardisation and quality of surgical procedures, though he was frequently hampered by administrative wrangling in the Surgeon General's office concerning levels of authority. Unfortunately, insufficient numbers of consultant surgeons were ever appointed to the Pacific campaigns where the demands for their expertise were probably greatest. In 1942, the European war consultants of the US Army were under the direction of the chief surgeon, Colonel (later Major-General) Paul R. Hawley. On only one known occasion was there such a violent difference of opinion between Hawley and a senior consultant that Hawley was forced to back down. He was described by one consultant as being:

> ... a superb chief in every respect. In addition to his excellent, but understandably not perfect ability to select men for important posts ... he was so often correct in his decisions that [others] were hard put to substantiate recommendations counter to his ideas.

Throughout 1943, there had been repeated efforts to standardise penicillin dosage, methods of debridement, the application of plaster-casts to wounded limbs and how to pack wounds that were left open for observation before later suturing. At the other end of the line of treatment back home, the reassignment and refurbishment of surgical and hospital resources on mainland America required time to prepare for receiving casualties from battlefronts in Europe, North Africa, the Mediterranean and the Pacific basin.

One reason for urgency was that many thousands of lives were being saved by the use of whole blood and plasma – how many will never be accurately known. As discussed earlier, plasma was more freely available and storable for much longer periods than whole blood. It kept casualties alive until whole blood was available and reconstructive surgery could proceed, whether it was in areas of war or safe back-up areas.

Among the standardised measures found essential to the survival of casualties with extensive compound fractures of the limbs (particularly lower) was the increasing use of the revolutionary Orr-Trueta technique[2] of enclosing the injured limb – after meticulous debridement and decompression of swollen muscles – within a full plaster cast. It was left in place for up to six weeks to allow healing of bone and soft tissues to occur uninterruptedly. Only intolerable odour, soiling or curiosity enforced earlier removal for inspection. The rigid cast allowed rapid transportation to more refined surgical care, usually undertaken in a long-leg Thomas splint. An adaptation was the 'Tobruk Splint' – the Thomas splint being also encased in plaster to facilitate rapid, more comfortable and less 'shocking' evacuation from the front.

These procedures were insisted on by consultants throughout all Allied armies after Dunkirk in 1940 and at Dieppe in 1942, and were highly developed in the later North and South Pacific campaigns with enormous salvage of both lives and limbs – especially with the advent of penicillin.

It was up to the surgical consultants to disseminate this information throughout the widely scattered theatres of war. By the time the hard fighting began in Europe and the Pacific, there was an 'average' use of more than one unit (roughly a pint) of whole blood for every casualty received in a treatment facility. The capability to collect blood on the American mainland and have it available within a few days of collection changed the face of resuscitation across every Allied battlefront. Consultants frequently found it necessary to

---

2. Winnett Orr was a US surgeon who first plastered severe civilian limb wounds in 1929 – a procedure refined by Joseph Trueta, a Spanish surgeon who had seen the German bombing injuries of civilians in the Spanish Civil War and then worked in exile in England, where he was ultimately appointed to the Nuffield Chair of Orthopaedics at Oxford in 1949. He also contributed to the understanding of acute kidney failure from shock, muscle damage and infection.

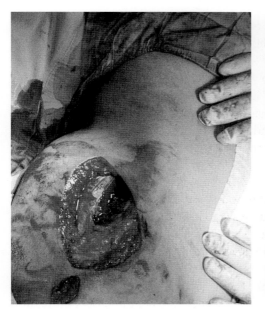
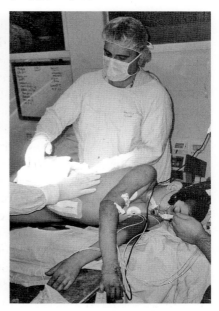

Above left: Massive shrapnel injury of the right hip, Second World War. Wounds were left open temporarily after removal of foreign bodies to allow drainage. (*US Army*)

Above right: Wound dressing applied loosely to allow observation. (*US Army*)

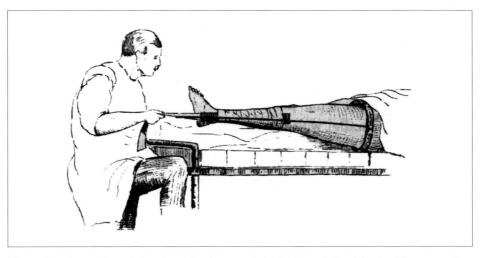

The tightening and straightening of a fractured thigh, immobilised in the Thomas splint. Encasing the leg and splint in plaster constitutes a 'Tobruk Splint'. (*Dr M. Crumplin*)

remind young surgeons to look for hidden areas of blood loss such as within the chest and abdomen and around fractures in the legs and pelvis. While resuscitation by transfusion in such cases accelerated fitness for surgery, once a patient was allowed to slip back into a shocked state because of inadequate blood replacement or a continuation of hidden bleeding, the chance of survival was greatly diminished.

A bonus for young surgeons was that whatever knowledge they gained from combat surgery prepared them for later management of serious civilian trauma – a benefit recognised by Hippocrates 2,000 years earlier. Surgeons also treated pre-existing civilian conditions that were detected for the first time when men went to war, as well as civilians in war areas, prisoners of war and the intermittent, non-combat illnesses and diseases of troops on both sides of battles.

Self-inflicted wounds – an ugly and inescapable association of all wars – were more likely to be detected by senior surgical consultants than by younger surgeons. Generous or naïve doctors might never make that diagnosis, but experienced surgeons were very aware of such wounds and the possibility of recurrence, however they were first treated. Most 'off-duty' bullet wounds were allegedly sustained while a man was allegedly 'cleaning his gun'. Other injuries were attributed to sporting accidents, chopping firewood or mishandling of weapons or hunting knives. These claims were often associated with psycho-neurotic illness or frank malingering and it required experience and very careful examination to reveal that they were not genuine injuries.

RUSSIAN MILITARY MEDICINE

Early in 1943, a Russian brigadier invited three British and three American surgeons to visit Russia, and Brigadier-General Elliott C. Cutler saw the opportunity for closer relationships between Allied medical services. It was arranged that, during such a visit, the American College of Surgeons and the English Royal College of Surgeons would confer honorary Fellowships on two famous Soviet surgeons: Professors Nikolai Burdenko and Serge Yudin.

From the outset, the Russians raised many irritating issues about protocol, including who would lead the mission to Russia and whether or not the visitors would wear uniform. Cutler was indifferent, but saw that there was an underlying agenda about which he could do nothing. The mission finally departed for Russia in full 'dress' uniform under Cutler's direction.

To start proceedings, the visitors were shown a Soviet motion picture depicting the care of wounded Soviet soldiers during evacuation from the front line up to the point of rehabilitation. Cutler's most striking observations were the frequent use of female troops in forward areas, the high standard of hygiene and the great value of air transport of the wounded. Other remarkable Russian innovations were also observed, such as the use of blood taken from cadavers for transfusion (half of it had to be discarded because of contamination by syphilis, tuberculosis or other bacteria) and a great reluctance to amputate arms.

There were many reminders that most frostbite actually occurred during the thawing of limbs and burns were infrequent except in air force personnel. The use of general anaesthesia was clearly inept (many patients were writhing in agony during surgical procedures) and there was a universal distaste for Professor Burdenko's oppressive influence on neurosurgery. He dictated policies throughout Russia, directing when, where, why, how and by whom surgery would be performed. The American and British were greatly impressed by the equivalent treatment of men and women in army service up to the rank of colonel. Off-duty nurses were frequently occupied in the construction of roads, houses and hospitals.

One morning the visitors were taken on an extensive sightseeing tour of Moscow and the Kremlin before the day ended with a special performance of *Swan Lake*. It came as a surprise to the Americans that letters of thanks and gifts could not be delivered directly to any Russian they met or admired without them first being scrutinised by a Russian officer.

On a tour of a laboratory renowned for its experiments with shock, the visitors saw techniques so crude that there had to be serious doubt about any conclusions drawn from them. When the visiting surgeons were gently sceptical of some surgical results claimed by the Russians, an unpleasant argument ensued. Finally, General Burdenko announced jovially that the visitors' comments were 'an example of how difficult it is to trust and negotiate with people who do not always bluntly state their views and positions'. Nonetheless, he ended the discussion with great joviality and a double hand-shake all round.

MILITARY ANAESTHESIA

It came as a surprise to the Senior American Consultant in Anesthesia, Ralph M. Tovell MD, when, more than twelve years after the end of the Second World War, he was asked to prepare an account of his war experience. Perhaps he felt some embarrassment at parts of the history he was to recall.

His first memory was of finding himself in the utter darkness of a dense London blackout in September 1942 with a US Army driver who was well able to traverse the busy streets confidently despite the conditions. For the consultant, Britain remained a confusing land where roads were blocked, directional signs were missing, citizens would give out no geographic information for security reasons and fog obscured the whole country during a long autumn.

As he was guided through military procedures and plans for deployment, he discovered a high level of anaesthetic expertise in some areas of the American service but very little in others. Almost all equipment was of British manufacture for which young American anaesthetists needed urgent orientation programmes. As an immediate stop-gap, anaesthetic nurses were rapidly recruited to develop surgical units where anaesthetists were in short supply. Many of them were retained permanently.

By June 1944, the consultant regarded his anaesthetic service as being competent for the needs of the D-Day invasion of Europe, but towards the end of that campaign he began to experience difficulty in providing adequate numbers of competent anaesthetists in forward units and evacuation hospitals. Apart from the shortage of new anaesthetists, those in service widely complained of 'battle fatigue'. So common was the syndrome that only younger men were sent to the most dangerous areas, while most of those over forty were confined to less challenging tasks in rear areas. They were the only medical group to shield their more-experienced men from the fighting front. Not surprisingly, their compatriots (surgeons, nurses and medics) found that very difficult to accept.

The problems of maintaining anaesthetic services became worse when the battle areas extended to southern France in 1944 and 1945. The severity of wounds had changed for the worse with the onset of winter and cold injuries becoming prevalent. Drug toxicity in cold weather was an increasing hazard when patients were warmed and rehydrated during treatment of shock. Normal doses of injected drugs such as morphine or pentothal could become 'locked-up' in cold tissues when blood circulation became too slow to wash them out. With improved blood flow after warming or when blood was replaced, drugs might be suddenly released into the general circulation at high concentration. Many complications and fatalities resulted until it was accepted that much smaller, repeated drug doses were better for shocked patients.

To compound the clinical problems, many anaesthetists felt they had been denied promotion in rank, despite long military service. They believed that they were being treated as second-class medical citizens and demanded incentives to maintain their enthusiasm. Others complained bitterly of being exhausted and overwhelmed by the burdens of casualties who often suffered injuries they had never seen before and scarcely understood. They certainly didn't want to be unduly concerned with them when the European war was almost won. Many nurses gladly undertook rapid training and, within a month or so, were able to take charge of whole anaesthetic sections and to conduct complex anaesthesia under difficult conditions. They were able to re-establish services even in the most demanding areas and earned the everlasting gratitude of the patients they anaesthetised. Of course, the surgeons, who had feared a complete interruption in some areas of their performance, were also grateful.

PERSONALITIES

Do everything you ask of those you command
Say what you mean
Mean what you say
Do not fear failure
Do more than is required of you
Do not take counsel of your fears
Always go forward
Take calculated risks
Give credit where it is due
Accept responsibility for the actions of yourself and your men.

– General George Patton, 1941

Those were rules of conduct for combat commanders recommended by General George Patton in 1941. Although they were directed at fighting men, according to Dr Michael E. DeBakey they were equally applicable to young surgeons who were newly appointed to war zones.

Colonel Elliott C. Cutler was one of the first and best regarded consultant surgeons appointed in the Second World War – initially in the European theatre. His wisdom and tenacity were reflected strongly in his diaries, but he did not get on well with Major-General Paul R. Hawley, Chief US Surgeon, probably due to friction over fine details. Although Hawley was critical of Cutler, a senior British consultant had nothing but praise for Cutler:

Perhaps no surgeon of the United States ever yearned or strove more earnestly to forge lasting bonds of friendship, not only between the surgeons, but between the peoples of the great English-speaking countries on either side of the North Atlantic and, to this end, he directed both written and spoken word.

Cutler was convinced of the need for consultants to work in peacetime on the same sorts of problems that they may encounter during war. During the First World War, he had appreciated better than many others that the consultants were an essential part of an efficient medical service. That was despite the problems of a triangular relationship between them, regular army officers and the much less experienced doctors who had come direct from civilian practice. Cutler was repeatedly preaching the obvious to the apathetic – that it was much too dangerous to wait for war before preparing a high-quality army medical service in peacetime:

We must practice lest we fail in our responsibility. What amount of labour by a doctor can equal the offer to his country of an infantryman, an aviator or any member of the fighting forces? There can be no demands upon [the doctors'] time and skill in peacetime … that our profession would not gladly give.

He had noticed that the British had wisely retained large numbers of consultants from the First World War in later peacetime posts and they were then effectively filling senior medical roles in the British Army. Obviously, Cutler was seriously discouraged when four surgical consultants left his service in 1943 with failing health. Some of them blamed the difficult circumstances under which they worked and criticised the intransigence of General Hawley. Looking back on Cutler's open annoyance, General Hawley spoke of him posthumously in somewhat qualified terms:

> … an innate honesty often compelled his professional judgements to be severe … his high ideals and devotion to duty made him, in his younger formative years, somewhat intolerant of mediocrity … the years brought him the wisdom that recognises the impossibility of universal perfection and a tolerance for human weakness … he required a lot of knowing … casual contact rarely revealed the true fineness of his character.

During 1943, Cutler had studied the use of sulphonamides and penicillin with the Australian researcher, Howard Florey. Although there was some doubt about the proper therapeutic place of the sulpha drugs, Cutler saw that their availability in the soldiers' kits provided great psychological benefits, whether or not those benefits could be demonstrated in a combat-wound setting. On the other hand, Cutler was increasingly impressed by penicillin as a life-saving drug, particularly in circumstances such as gas gangrene and other serious infections of bones, abdominal wounds and open head injuries.

COLD INJURY

Military records suggest that, apart from Napoleon's armies in 1812, no military force had ever experienced so many and such severe 'cold injuries' as those seen in Russia by the Germans, or by the Allies in Italy in 1944–45. The latter were enough to threaten the overall efficiency of military operations in Europe. The 1943–44 reports of American surgical consultants emphasised the hazard but they were not acted on for a year. Very little of the British experience of the First World War, the American experience of the bleakly-cold and wet Aleutian Island campaigns of 1942 or the lessons of the Mediterranean campaigns of the Second World War had been transferred to the European theatre. There were over 70,000 cases of trench foot admitted to hospital in the autumn and winter of 1944–45 alone – 5 per cent of all admissions.

By the end of the Second World War, nearly 100,000 US troops had been disabled by cold injuries. Worst of all, they proved difficult to treat and carried a high rate of significant permanent impairment. Fortunately, cold injuries to hands tended to be less common and less severe than those affecting feet. Troops in poor physical condition or with a past history of chilblains, 'poor circulation' or slow heart rates seemed more susceptible. Tobacco smokers were probably also at greater risk because of the constricting effect of nicotine on small blood vessels, but for unknown reasons, possibly for morale, they were not prohibited from smoking when other measures for avoidance were thought more important.

It was not as though frostbite was something new. It had been mentioned in the ancient writings of Hippocrates, Aristotle and Galen. French surgeons wrote about it in the Napoleonic Wars and it had been taken very seriously in the American Civil War. The penalty paid was the loss of toes, fingers, hands or feet. Fortunately, ground-level injury rarely occurred above the ankle or wrist. The tragedy was that troops took the initial discomfort lightly because it was often mild. It was only when they warmed themselves before a fire that painful thawing occurred and gangrene progressed rapidly.

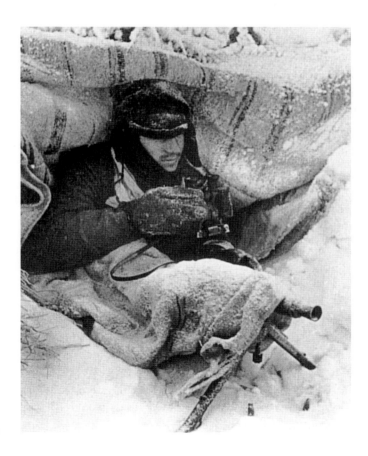

A soldier at great risk from freezing conditions in Europe.

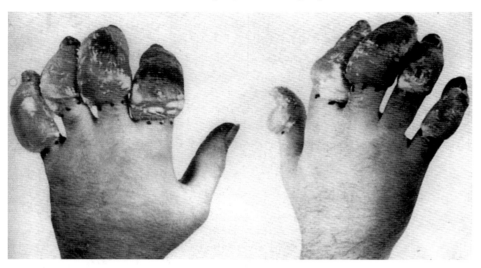

The results of ground-level frostbite with lines of demarcation of dead tissue marked by spots. (*Dr M. E. DeBakey*)

Consultants needed to urgently standardise the approach to all forms of cold injury, such as immersion foot, trench foot, shelter foot and frost bite. All had the same vascular pathology arising from prolonged exposure to a variable ratio of cold and moisture. Every layer of the terrestrial military organisation, in particular the infantry who were at greatest risk, required education in the problem. Foot hygiene, warm and dry socks, protective footwear and adequate rest periods became essential care for all concerned.

The US 8th Air Force was also slow to recognise that high altitude cold injury had essentially the same pathology as ground-level injury, the only difference being that the ground-type included moisture.

A great cost resulted from failures to learn from past experience. The extensive British experience of cold injury in the First World War had not been exploited in planning in the Second World War and had not carried over to the Korean War in 1950. To make matters worse, it was found necessary in the Italian autumn of 1944 to give priority to transporting fuel and ammunition rather than winter clothing for troops, resulting in many more potentially avoidable injuries.

Sir John Monash had risen to command all Australian divisions on the Western Front at the end of the First World War and had been especially concerned with cold injury occurring at ground level. To that end, he improvised laundries and drying facilities to enable his troops to have dry gloves, socks and underwear at least twice weekly. In addition, wherever possible, he insisted on a hot meal being delivered to his men on the front line, even in the midst of battle. Much that had been learned from Monash and

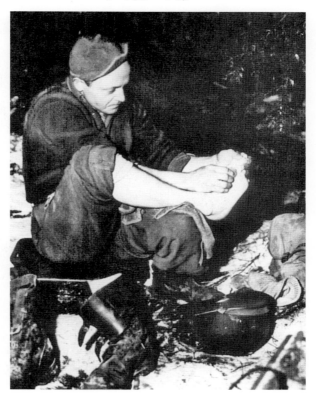

Changing into dry socks,
Second World War.
(*Dr M. E. DeBakey*)

others in the First World War had to be re-learned at enormous cost to soldiers and their surgeons during the Second World War.

After such dismal failures, Colonels T. F. Whayne and M. E. DeBakey were commissioned to write a definitive document on cold injury for the Medical Department of the US Army, published in 1958. Their classic study emphasised that there had been no excuses for its high frequency and that it was possible to prevent most cases with proper precautions, education and, above all, discipline. It is a tragedy that this brilliant exposition took so long to be commissioned and publicised. Russian armies operated in regions of extreme cold and were well acquainted with cold injury and the means of avoiding it. They wore loose, warm clothing and fur gloves. Their large boots came in only three sizes and were of soft, pliable felt without heels or seams. They didn't bother with socks, but troops were supplied with bandages of linen or woollen cloth which they wrapped around their feet until they snugly fitted their boots.

Wet bandages were immediately removed and reversed with the dry portions from the top placed around the feet. They sometimes added newspaper wrapping to increase protection. No soldier was permitted to sleep until his feet and footwear had been inspected. Russia regarded cold injury as a

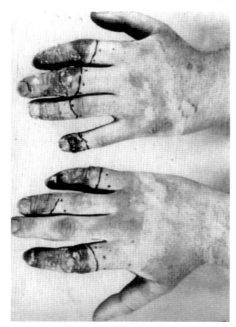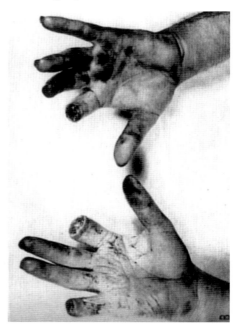

Above left and right: High-altitude hand injuries without moisture component, demarcating and some amputations. (*Dr M. E. DeBakey*)

preventable condition for which the responsibility lay with everybody from the individual up to the chief surgeon. Any or all of those ranks could be severely punished for neglect of safe care.

For all surgeons, it was a frustrating and difficult problem. Even when amputation seemed inevitable, great consideration was required to judge how radical it should be. However the injuries were managed, even where men returned to service, there was an average loss of three months' service per patient, amounting to a total of some 25,000 years of lost time in the Second World War. Many would never return to full service and the worst were disabled for life from amputations.

VALUE OF SURGICAL ASSIGNMENTS

The experience of the US Army in Europe taught many valuable lessons for future Allied administrations. One of them concerned the allocation of surgical personnel to various posts. The issue was addressed by Colonel Cutler in the following terms:

> Evacuation hospitals carry a very responsible load; the brunt of initial surgery of the wounded falls upon them. Eyes, limbs and lives will be sacrificed

unnecessarily unless surgery of the highest quality is performed in them. In the field, the surgical consultant does not have sufficient leeway or reserves of personnel to correct staffing errors. An Army in combat never has a reserve of medical officers. To the contrary, it always has a deficit. Deficits in field hospitals can be covered by auxiliaries but the evacuation hospitals must take care of their own personnel problems. They must be staffed, therefore, with the greatest care. Errors in staffing were not always easy to correct once the army hospital was located overseas.

In a nine-month period from August 1944 to May 1945, the hospitals and clearing stations of the 7th US Army alone admitted 61,000 'wounded', 27,000 'non-combat wounded' (including general surgical, orthopaedic, motor vehicle and self-inflicted injuries) and 100,000 with 'non-combat diseases'. The last category included pre-existing abnormalities, infections and psychiatric conditions. Very few in any category died in a hospital or clearing station. Definitions and details of non-combat 'wounds' and 'diseases' are difficult to discover, but many were probably of civilian type. In early 1943, the Chief US Consultant in Surgery in the European Theatre of Operations stated explicitly that the British orthopaedic surgeons' view – that they were best able to look after general trauma – was absurd:

> [They] ... cannot care for trauma of the head, or care for the ruptured kidney or ruptured spleen, nor would [they] have any idea of what to do with non-perforating thoracic injury ... a disturbing finding in England is that only orthopaedic surgeons [are expected to] treat fractures and other forms of trauma. This seems to me to create a grave danger in the broad outlook of medical practice, both for the people we treat and for the profession.

The great German blitzes on Britain had revealed that fractures were not well treated by the 'ordinary' doctor and somebody had decided that only orthopaedic surgeons should treat them in future. Senior Americans believed that this would leave Britain with too few surgeons able to treat fractures and its younger surgeons would have almost no experience of treating any form of trauma during their surgical education. Had Britain trained their young doctors adequately, '... she would now have thousands of people trained in trauma and not just a pitiful handful'. These were strong and unpalatable criticisms, but the British realised the urgency of the situation and rapidly remedied the problem.

At that time, the Chief US Surgical Consultant, the Surgeon General and their British counterparts saw fit to re-issue iron-clad directives to all surgical staff about gas gangrene that had followed premature wound closure without first carrying out thorough cleansing and drainage. They thundered:

Primary suture of all wounds of the extremities under war conditions is NEVER to be done. It is permitted only after debridement in certain abdominal, chest and facial injuries. It is STRICTLY FORBIDDEN that any compound fracture or extensive wound of the extremities be treated with closure of the wound ... [or that] amputation be done higher than [ideal] ... commanding officers will be held responsible for abandonment of the improper procedures described above and the necessary instruction and compliance with these directives.

Given the rigidity in this order, it was inevitable that the Chief Consultant soon found it necessary to qualify his views with simple examples:

... previously healthy and clean, vigorous young men reach a hospital within two hours of injury, thus simulating civilian hospital practice. Several have had to have immediate amputation and, in selected cases, short-flap amputation has permitted early secondary closure and even primary closure with highly satisfactory results. There should be a difference in therapy according to terrain and environment. Thus, a sailor knocked into the sea by a shell fragment and immediately picked up and taken to a hospital ship,

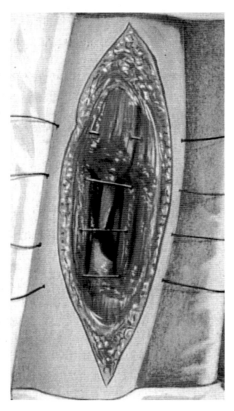

Open compound fracture with delayed suture closure and observation. (*Dr M. Crumplin*)

and an aviator wounded in clean clothes in a clean airplane and reaching a hospital within three hours, and a wounded infantry soldier who has lived in a foxhole, covered with mud and clothed in filthy garments for weeks and who reaches a hospital in six to twelve hours, [all] need entirely different treatment at the hands of the surgeon.

Such dogma reflected the need to have uniform attitudes among a huge army of medical personnel who had varied backgrounds, and were spread over many sites. The concept of 'do not suture' was never meant to encourage undue delay in wound closure, or to leave the responsibility for the timing of wound closure to somebody else to worry about later. In fact, yet another comment from medical command contained a major retraction that allowed surgeons to use their discretion. Given the variable conditions of combat, the advice was sensible and explicit, 'Not to suture a wound initially is good practice. To fail to close it at the first safe moment is neglecting an opportunity to protect the soldier against further infection and loss of function'.

A subject of much discussion between surgeons towards the end of the war concerned the use of Landing Ship Tanks (LSTs) – or similar craft – for the evacuation of wounded men from beaches. One British general believed that an LST was a 'cold, dirty trap' and completely unsuitable for the job. Others thought that serious injuries of the chest and abdomen should be treated urgently on an LST rather than waiting for evacuation to a distant location and risking death in transit. Neither view was recommended by high command, but it was agreed that, 'If a man happens to be qualified to operate [on patients aboard an LST], good. If not, he [would] have to depend upon [giving] morphine.'

But one senior surgeon was much less enthusiastic:

[Most of] ... these surgeons are young chaps – recent graduates. They will not have done any kind of [surgical] residency. Operate on a patient's belly on an LST? The real question is whether it is better to operate BEFORE leaving the shore and then put [the soldier] immediately on an LST.

The issue was never resolved and the crucial decisions were finally left, as always, to the senior surgeon in a particular situation and location.

During the landing of Allied forces at Normandy in June 1944, an unidentified combat surgeon wrote of his personal experience:

... [I] ordered 50 billion units of penicillin ... only 600 million now here ... half on beaches, half on LSTs and the rest for distribution here ... but it is a mess ... all of us asked for lots of penicillin. We order and none comes. The Continental invasion is on at last ... all are excited ... saw bad case blown up on ship ... left foot gone, open fracture of right leg into knee joint ... very ill ...

[wound] not yet dressed at six days ... bad treatment but not yet infected ... have had five or six cases of gas gangrene ... not all amputations, yet six days old! Why no more infection? Sulphonamides and penicillin? [We] ... saw a German with a right lower-quarter abdominal wound ... the prisoner said, 'We Germans have no chance. Replacements are not allowed.'

At that frenetic time, the US Chief Surgeon again saw fit to repeat his cautions about wound management:

If every medical officer in the first week devoted himself [only] to the control of haemorrhage, adequate dressing, adequate treatment of shock with plasma and blood, and perfect immobilisation [of the fractures], a perfect task would have been performed. I would suggest less immediate surgery and more emphasis on properly evacuating those who can travel safely.

Given the general high regard for stretcher-bearers in combat, it is very surprising that a British surgeon at Normandy spoke critically of first aid and triage:

Treatment at their level is not particularly skilful. It is a mixture of commonsense and humanity. If they would only use commonsense and stick to a routine treatment. Simplification is what we want. They have to get the patients out, but they must get them out successfully treated so that nothing happens. They must give first-aid medical treatment to get [the soldier] back, in at least no worse shape than he started ... the surgeons must learn the type of case they can treat in forward hospitals or the type they must send on [to more capable hospitals]. Anything the surgeon can send on saves effort [at the front]. Surgery in forward areas should be very limited. A mediocre [surgeon] may be much more valuable than a good surgeon who is going to complicate things by [aggressively] treating every case he sees.

Such petulant comments might be interpreted in various ways, but they strongly suggest that the stretcher-bearers were being blamed for problems that were not their prime responsibility.

MANAGING THE PACIFIC BASIN

The Normandy surgeon's comments probably reflected insoluble problems in his area, but they were worse elsewhere. There seems no doubt that the surgical results achieved by inexperienced surgeons in the Pacific War were generally inferior to those of surgeons in the European, Mediterranean and North African theatres. Colonel F. T. Hallam, a surgeon in the Solomon Islands, wrote:

War neurosis starts with the poor officer who cracks up; then the men go; most of nature's creatures here are harmless, except for man; flies get in your mouth but mosquitoes are very rare – there are red ants in the area but they don't bother much. Some masks have been found that were used by the Japanese for terrorising purposes – this climate is hot and wet, everything moulds, including the feet, no wonder fungus infection is a problem – here is one place where folks don't want to wear medals or discs or anything else to distinguish themselves – everybody from the General on down wants to be as inconspicuous as possible.

By the time the Pacific campaigns were under way, surgical resources were stretched far beyond what had ever been expected. Besides, many medical solutions did not become available until consultants could begin to standardise treatment and disseminate best principles of practice to every operating surgeon, wherever he was. The wet, humid conditions of much of the Pacific suddenly reintroduced problems of gas gangrene. Yet again, it was necessary to acquaint troops and medical officers with the same aspects of foot-care as had been clearly established earlier in the northern hemisphere. To make matters worse, there was great concern about the high rates of complications and mortality when anaesthetics were given by unskilled anaesthetists. In an attempt to boost those services, crash-programmes to train nurses in anaesthesia were re-instituted in many battle zones. History shows that they filled that role with great expertise. As a result of these emergency practices of the Second World War, in rural areas of the US today some 70 per cent of all anaesthetics are given by nurses. It was left to surgical consultants to evaluate needs and assign surgical and anaesthetic personnel throughout the Western Pacific. Those campaigns could not have succeeded without nurses being able to manage the demands for anaesthetists, which continued until Japan's surrender. The reason why a consultant in anaesthesia was never appointed to the Western Pacific is unknown, but a poor compromise towards the war's end was to have general advice from a naval anaesthetist headquartered in Manila. Perhaps the specialist nurse anaesthetists had filled requirements so well that they averted a potential crisis. That meant that there was a less pressing need for a consultant to closely oversee operations.

Because of the aggressive attitude of the Japanese towards hospitals and prisoners, many medical personnel were trained for the first time in the use of small arms for personal protection, though few used them.

By early 1945, major preparations for the invasion of Japan were underway and massive casualties were expected. Newly arrived medical officers in the Western Pacific were generally less experienced than those in earlier campaigns and required intensive education in the essential elements of battle care. Shocking films of casualties in earlier battles were shown repeatedly to all medical staff to prepare them for what were expected to be the last, violent days of the Pacific War. In the educational phase, the value of surgical consultants was paramount. They were the essential experts the army needed to integrate and maximise its surgical capabilities.

Colonel A. W. Oughterson, MC, a senior surgeon from New York, was assigned to the Pacific in mid-1943 and ultimately served in every major centre of that campaign. Like Colonel Elliott Cutler in Europe, he was a brilliant surgeon and teacher. Both were men of ideas who were impatient to have them translated into action, and both were frequently critical of complex command structures. In today's misleading parlance, both men probably fitted the description of the 'disruptive' doctor who is indispensable in grave circumstances.

Chief among Oughterson's concerns was the slow evacuation of serious casualties, which took only hours over the relatively short distances of Europe, but in the huge distances of the Pacific area, could take days or weeks. To make matters worse, tropical diseases such as malaria were endemic in the Pacific, and gas gangrene, which had been bad enough in Europe, was even more frequent with the moist earth of tropical islands laden with excreta and dangerous bacteria.

The views of Cutler and Oughterson corresponded remarkably in their principles of casualty management. Each Pacific island was a unit in itself, reliant on the talent of medical staff located there. Oughterson constantly pleaded for more qualified surgeons to be placed well forward in combat areas to limit delays in access to specialist standards of care. He had '... never seen a surgeon who did good surgery back home, do bad surgery in the army'. He commented frequently on the principal cause of war neurosis – unhappy, idle soldiers who had doubts about the expertise of their surgical carers. It seems there was some reason for the surgical concern.

Oughterson's successor complained that younger and less talented medical officers, working in the most unfavourable conditions, were not given as much credit by him as they deserved, especially when they were already 'giving everything they had'. There is abundant evidence in Oughterson's diaries to show that this was an unjustified criticism. He clearly recognised his surgeons' immaturity, but attributed recurrent problems solely to their much too rapid training and their slow enlistment. When he took over the South-West Pacific consultancy, Oughterson was well aware that there were too few experienced surgeons available to teach younger men and, in any case, the breadth of the Pacific basin made regular supervision difficult or impossible.

Never before was a mobile consultant such an essential surgical element in maintaining an army. His meticulously maintained diaries between August 1943 and August 1945 carry an astonishing range of surgical wisdom joined to his superb skills as an administrator. He accepted without complaint the personal burden of extensive, uncomfortable travel among widely dispersed operations. His diary entries about the many hundreds of inspections he conducted in those two years, much abbreviated here, speak for themselves. Every word demonstrates what responsibility and surgical care meant to him. Few men could maintain a programme as arduous as this:

> Left at 0730 hrs and arrived in Noumea 1400 hrs, quartered at The Grand Hotel Central which I am told was formerly a house of ill-repute – inspected medical supply situation (we are fighting the Japs, not each other) – visited a hospital, poor site, daily records fair, no monthly records – good equipment – having trouble with skin-tight plaster casts.

With that, Oughterson finished his first report. At 2 a.m. on the following morning he travelled to Espiritu Santo in the New Hebrides to inspect the evacuation hospital that was receiving many casualties with dirty wounds, but had very few orthopaedic infections. He went on to Guadalcanal to confer with senior surgeons and generals and observed landing ships unloading 200 patients at a time onto the beach, most of them wounded more than three days earlier. He saw that better facilities were needed on the landing craft and reported the need for a 500-bed hospital with facilities capable of increasing that number:

> Up at 0330 hrs and left for the Solomons – took off over some of the worst roads I have ever seen, with four fighter escorts overhead – talked to the colonel in charge – a fine person doing a grand job – he needs more help to do it. – Drove through a devastated area pitted with Japanese foxholes – 5,000 of them were here – it took three divisions to get them out – many Japanese skeletons lying about in their clothes – clearing stations here function as surgical or field hospitals – too much diarrhoea here – must look into the sedation employed – anti-toxin for gas gangrene plentiful – chest wounds well handled – hospital surrounded by barbed wire on which [rattling] tin cans have been placed [to warn of approaching] Japanese who have raided the hospital – war here appears to be more vicious than in other places – the trail for jeeps and ambulances is very rough – some with severe fractures die as a result of the ride – boats have regular schedules for stopping along the shore to [collect and] transport the wounded.

There he found the mud was knee deep and the weather hot and steamy. The roads were almost impassable, the food was of inferior quality, equipment was in short supply and most of the doctors were young and inexperienced but being rotated out of action every few months – far too often to maintain competence. They lacked oxygen supplies, a gasoline-fuelled mechanical washing machine and a refrigerator for blood products. No one there was able to repair broken spectacles. The wounded were being evacuated from as far as 5 miles away, sometimes through contaminated swamps and streams.

He saw less war neurosis than in other areas – a fact he attributed to better leadership:

> Elsewhere, I found six or eight tents knocked down by 500-pound bombs and eight men killed – why not have a little more [insect] screening in order to protect the food? – the flies swarm but diarrhoea not a great problem here yet – many wounds are infected here by arriving late – instruments are kept in sterilising solutions such as alcohol – evacuation is a problem – lack of organisation results in many delays – can this movement be correlated with the navy? – not enough good surgeons available for operating while on landing craft.
>
> The morale of this outfit is low; the old problems of [unfairness in] rotation and promotion – many ear infections and eye problems but no optometry – need for sulpha drugs for dressings – one month is considered too long a period to keep men in the line – they may have only three hot meals during that time – they get little sleep and they must fight all day – it takes a superman – malingering is not high here – the psychiatrist says that neuro-psychiatric cases are either "those who have had trauma, or those that are afraid of trauma" – efficiency is dropping rapidly.

Oughterson had a mixed experience on Guadalcanal. On one occasion he saw a boat load of Americans who looked more like pirates than soldiers. One man responded to an order by lying down and saying 'I don't know or give a damn' and went back to sleep through a bombing attack. He found poor equipment and even a lack of batteries and light bulbs. He questioned whether debridement was being done adequately. Malaria was widespread and there were few dental facilities. Everybody was asking for better insect screening. He met one of the finest commanding officers of his experience on Guadalcanal. They had treated more than twenty cases of gangrene during the month of July.

Oughterson suggested that more and better debridement should be done in forward areas and reinforced the need for adequate splinting of fractures and adequate control of haemorrhage. A further problem was a lack of detailed 'tags' attached to patients to tell the next surgeon what had been done, and when and what complications were expected. Peripherally, he repeatedly saw poor initial wound management with cases of premature closure of wounds. All of these factors were compounded by protracted delays before the wounded could reach a major hospital:

> A boy was riding on the fender of a truck when a bullet from a machine-gun, one of ours, hit him in the back – he was instantly paralysed – this happened at 1700 hrs – he arrived by plane at hospital at noon next day. Another boy, the tail gunner in a B-24 on a bombing mission on Bougainville, parachuted

from his burning plane and was strafed by the Japs – he was shot through the belly on the right side and had a large exit wound just to the right of his spine – there were six perforations of the intestine and the missile had passed near his right kidney – he was operated on within two and a half hours and is doing well this afternoon.

Another boy, a gunner on a bomber, was shot through the upper third of the left leg ... both major blood vessels were cut and there was a complicated fracture – amputation was necessary, done within a few hours and he is doing well – air transport of the sick can accomplish wonders but it does not replace proper surgical care close to the place of injury – a detonated dud hurt no-one [troops] but a cook 200 yards away in the mess hall stopped the fragments – took out both eyes and the bridge of his nose – he is in good condition and wants to know about his eyesight – they need well qualified specialist surgeons in the forward areas.

On the next leg of his journey, Oughterson travelled very early to arrive in Espiritu Santo at 10.30 a.m. He saw a wounded soldier who should have been evacuated promptly but had been unnecessarily delayed for twenty-four hours and by then had developed gangrene. It was typical of his attention to detail that he also reported the need for better litters and hob-nailed boots for the stretcher-bearers to enable them to walk more safely in mud. Overall, surgery in Santo was better than in many other areas, although sanitation needed to be improved and malaria control was overwhelmed. Transportation was a continuing challenge and he was disturbed to find so many young surgeons placed in posts for which they were not qualified.

He objected strenuously to the proposition that most head, chest and belly wounds were fatal whatever treatment was given and should therefore not be pursued. That attitude, he felt, would destroy morale and a more aggressive surgical attitude was needed. He learned that the Japanese were using American casualties as bait in ambushes. He suggested that men be instructed to crawl for cover rather than remain upright when wounded and also recommended green wound-dressings rather than white which attracted attention. He believed a good dose of morphine was essential in every man's kit and that sulpha drugs lowered fevers.

At one point he encountered a public servant on inspection from the Surgeon General's office who walked unannounced into his room with a troop of senators. One of them suggested that troops should not be allowed to self-medicate with morphine and sulpha drugs. Oughterson replied that he regarded that as a hasty and dangerous suggestion and that such decisions were best left to him and other consultants:

Arose at 0300 hrs and arrived Fiji at 1430 hrs – shortages of various sorts of equipment and need to categorise hospitals and surgeons according to

their capabilities so that the wounded are directed appropriately and quickly
– there are 2,500 beds at Fiji and too much medical and surgical talent not
fully occupied – another 2,000 beds could be made available so long as well
organised transfer of the worst cases can be accomplished rapidly and treated
better than elsewhere – shortage of anaesthetists – too many high ranking
officers have been promoted without proper professional qualifications –
some old Army men look more to their organisations than to the good of the
service – the area surgeon does not feel free to move these men about – there
are just not enough qualified men to go round.

In New Caledonia men with simple ailments are being evacuated and those
with more serious injuries requiring expert care are staying put – psychotic
patients are being given a physical diagnosis which makes treatment more
difficult – I see a dirty hospital, hot and on low-mosquito ridden grounds
– left for Santo again on naval flying-boat, next visited Guadalcanal again
– discussed matters of supply of various equipment – prophylactic kits
[condoms] still being used with no females within 1,000 miles of here, so
they are used as covers for pistol barrels, watches and pocket drug kits –
what good are mops with no floors to mop? – generators are needed urgently
after eleven were lost – we are equipping to invade Bougainville – convoy
escorts firing on Japanese lines – tremendous confusion on shore until we
found the clearing station and collecting station – the sky suddenly seemed
full of Japanese aircraft.

After six hours of bombing and strafing during one night, Oughterson made it
a practice to hang his jungle hammock in a fox-hole for safer sleeping. Noting
that the Japanese had been shooting at a marines' hospital, Oughterson
instructed his surgical staff and soldiers to shoot anything that moved outside
the area. A favourite Japanese tactic was to climb trees at night and await
sniping opportunities in the morning when there were people moving about
the hospital. He approved the fact that Americans with carbines were having
target practice with the tree dwellers. Over and over again, he noted that
junior surgeons were treating patients who required greater expertise than
they were receiving. Disturbingly, there had been serious conflict between
the scarce senior surgeons at first-aid stations where over-confident juniors
lacked understanding of complex issues. His next report emphasised yet again
that surgeons could not be held responsible for good surgery without quality
equipment and that clearing stations could not be expected to turn out first-
class work without first-class surgeons. There was little else that he could do
but report the deficiencies. However, it seemed he received poor, if any, support
from his high command:

On Bougainville, great progress – many stories of bombing, strafing and
shelling – eight cases of gas gangrene – several patients died in transit – much

shelling by Japanese – raining constantly – a lot of discussion about how to keep the doctors happy while they are in the service – the consensus is that it is generally impossible unless they are busy and successful.

Guadalcanal on 7 December, remembering it is two years today since Pearl Harbor – more talk about need for thorough debridement to avoid gas gangrene [being] seen in about ten per cent of compound fractures – many inadequately cleaned up – off to Noumea tomorrow – expecting a bumpy ride because of the storms – pleased to be promoted to full Colonel today – mobile surgical hospitals on the way – will they have qualified surgeons?

In Fiji – met General George Marshall – saw an operating team four feet underground – some surgeons are wondering why they have been here for three years without relief – island hopping to Bougainville, then Santo again – psychiatric disturbances may be due to Atebrin [preventative for malaria] – the wounded have a bad time because litter bearers take ten hours to bring them in through the jungle, eight men per litter – leaving for Guadalcanal tomorrow without a fighter escort – one plane recently disappeared with all on board – everyone must wear lifebelts – plenty of bugs – one commander says: "No [doctor] should control a unit here which comes from his home town because few people can be really objective in that situation, particularly if they have to go back to the town to live [together]" – much praise for various commanders because of their excellent work, control, organisation and standards – I find some of this depressing – probably need some leave.

His next stop was Bougainville, where he toured the front lines and saw 400 Japanese dead being buried by American bulldozers. It was the enemy's practice to walk safely across a minefield by stepping on the bodies of their own men who had been killed by detonating mines. No prisoners were being taken by either side. One hospital was located near a battery of Japanese artillery, around which lay 1,300 Japanese dead. Clearing stations were being shelled daily. One attack hit the local surgeon's office, but he was lucky enough to be absent at the time. Japanese hand grenades were generally considered fairly innocuous because their charge was small. Oughterson's overall recommendation was that a 750-bed evacuation hospital was needed to allow eight functioning operating tables with thirty or forty patients being resuscitated from shock in adjacent rooms. He did not say if that suggestion was ever taken up:

All is worsened by being transferred long distances – many cases of ruptured ear drums from blast, some men not knowing it had occurred – another had defective vision and had shot at his own men in mistake – awaiting heavy barrage from Japanese – morale high though quite a few psychiatric cases – most of them had some trouble before entering the Army – the morale of those serving overseas, both medical and infantry, is in inverse correlation to the income of similar people back home; if the income of the civilian population were limited to the corresponding army [income], this factor would be eliminated.

The 37th is the 'Banner Division' of the South Pacific – better supplies and faster delivery still required in forward areas – all men need a second pair of spectacles – foxholes have to be deeper and narrower and [men should] crawl more often to avoid being hit in silhouette – citations for medics are insufficient, some taking more risks than the infantry – severe chest wounds carrying up to 30 per cent mortality if requiring operation – more flame throwers are needed for defence against mass attacks – I have a lot of reports to finish for Washington – ordered to go to New Zealand, then Noumea, then Hawaii – asked to write a report on the function of consulting surgeons.

While critical of some of the portable surgical hospitals with inadequate staffing, a visiting general observed that, "I didn't know your standards would be so high!"

The anaesthetists are scattered all over the place, some doing executive work when they should be giving anaesthetics – still labouring at educational directives to make management details uniform – battling inadequate staffing or inefficient distribution of good staff.

He found a well-run, 500-bed hospital on Maui with plenty of experienced nurses. They were expecting a large number of casualties from the Philippines where invasion was planned and he hoped to get feedback from treated soldiers about the quality of their care. He complained sorely about having to write long-winded reports about trivial matters and having his most important reports ignored with little or no explanation. He sensed resentment about his repeated requests and recommendations. He again reported of inadequate specialist appointments in all areas of complex surgery and of having no established anaesthetic department headed by competent doctors. In effect, he was an unwelcome 'whistle blower':

Left today for Guam where there is a 750-bed hospital 20 miles from the port but close to the airfields – should be able to take patients in a couple of weeks – many more nurses required here – evacuation of injured men still too slow – saw a landing ship which is the finest medical unit afloat, converted to a 200-bed hospital ship, doing excellent work with good laboratories – five surgeons and 18 medics on board each landing ship, functioning as floating emergency hospitals – some attempts to bomb them.

In the Philippines, many blood banks functioning well but much more blood necessary – difficulties from lack of refrigeration and ice – heavy losses of men from the front line, some having to be transferred 1,500 miles to the nearest established hospital – the South Pacific area has 45,000 hospital beds in 23 general hospitals – the Japanese attempted an invasion by paratroops leading to an all-night fight – none of the hospital personnel had training in firearms other than shooting squirrels – that needs correction – the prima-donnas and the weak egos undoubtedly retard military accomplishment – in the army, as in civilian life, if non-medical men are to assume administrative responsibilities for medical care, they should be educated in medical problems, at least to the extent of being able to identify a competent surgeon – General MacArthur's quarters are huge and beautifully furnished.

He saw many casualties resulting from Japanese bombardment. Again there was evidence of inadequate initial wound treatment and many soldiers who could have returned to duty quickly had, instead, been rapidly evacuated – a complete aberration of sensible triage. He found the roads crowded with natives fleeing from combat areas and a deafening roar of guns and screeching of shells arose from a fleet of battleships firing from both sides of where he sheltered.

It was a similar situation at all the beaches. Many landing craft were serving as surgical operating platforms. There was plenty of well-refrigerated blood available from the American mainland as well as troop donors. He visited Guam again en route to Hawaii before returning to the Philippines. He bitterly described the huge gulf between his philosophy of good surgical care and what he was experiencing:

> Get the right man at the right place at the right time, with adequate numbers and adequate equipment – none of this can be accomplished without planning – consultants in the Pacific have not been consulted in planning – like trying to lock the stable door after the horse has gone – the consultant has little left for him to do sometimes – skilled surgeons should be in the forward areas where the worst problems exist.

He later described political issues and events:

> ... excellent hospitals on Iwo Jima – reviewing the need for a civilian medical care in Manila where most of 5,000 beds are already occupied – again short of personnel – trench foot a continuing problem regardless of telling soldiers how to manage it – Japan turned down our surrender terms today [27 July 1945] – most betting the war will end within three months. Asked to board a Japanese hospital ship intercepted nearby by a destroyer flotilla – we hear that the Japanese have accepted the Potsdam Ultimatum – much contraband on the hospital ship – 1,600 Japanese on board sleeping on and among large quantities of arms and ammunition – no seriously ill patients – all able to walk off the ship and later examined, some with malnutrition – no wounded, generally regarded as slightly ill.
>
> August 13, 1945 – peace seems near – the Japanese have accepted an ultimatum following the atomic bombs. [They put] the responsibility for

destroying civilisation upon the United States. The Japanese Emperor's announcement to the population suggested that he felt no remorse and had no intention of changing his views about Japan's role in the Pacific War when he told his people: 'The enemy has used a new and cruel bomb ... and to continue would have been the total extinction of human civilisation. Such being the case, how are we to return ourselves before the hallowed spirits of our ancestors? By working to save and maintain the structure of the Imperial State. Unite your total strength ... so you may enhance the glory of the Imperial State.'

Oughterson's diary finished with a simple summary:

We have gained a military decision, not their ultimate defeat ... boarded an army transport ship today with orders to pack within 24 hours ... off to Tokyo.

In Tokyo he participated in a joint allied commission investigating the effects of the atomic bomb on Japan and edited its formal report. He described how more than 100,000 persons, including senior surgical consultants, had been involved in three years of preparation for the invasion of Japan when an American bomber, christened *Enola Gay*, dropped a bomb and finished the war. It exploded 500 metres above the city of Hiroshima at 8.15 a.m. on 6 August 1945. A few days later, a similar bomb was exploded over a shipyard at Nagasaki. The stark political effect of the atom bombs was to persuade the Japanese government to think the unthinkable and surrender – without acknowledging defeat.

Despite the casualties they caused, the bombs undoubtedly brought forward a release from the agony of violence and attrition pervading Japanese cities and much of the South-West Pacific region at that time. Many more civilians had already died in the conventional bombing of Japan than from atom bombs. The immediate medical challenge for both sides was the occurrence of a massive blast followed by thermal and nuclear radiation within a mile of the

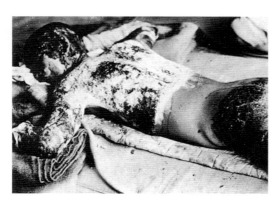

Severe burns from atomic explosion, Hiroshima, 1945. Extensive internal damage might also occur. (*US Army*)

explosions. As always expected by those involved, there was little or nothing that could be done for most of those affected.

Before he retired from the Pacific theatre, Oughterson was asked to examine Japanese prisoners of war in the Philippines. He found most of them undernourished, anaemic and wasted. Infection and gangrene were common and splints were crude and ineffective. Despite their later supervision by US Army surgeons, Japanese medical officers showed a general lack of experience and judgement.

NOTES ON REHABILITATION

The theory in the First World War had been that, when a man's physical wounds had healed, time and rest would usually bring him back to 'normal' – sooner or later. Whether or not Post Traumatic Stress Disorder (PTSD) was clearly defined, well managed or ever recoverable, some formulae achieved remarkable results when applied intensively in locations remote from combat.

Early in the Second World War, the US Air Force astounded the rehabilitation world by declaring that very little time was actually required to return injured men to duty if the victim's attention was totally and powerfully directed into a creative programme of mental and physical activity. The idea was based on an old concept of troops helping themselves. Many doubted it could be as simple as that.

Patients were provided with educational material and made to keep records of their rate of recovery. They selected their own convalescent activities and were assigned to a doctor who became their close personal physician. They also had a physical therapist, a psychiatrist and other medical specialists as necessary. Among the triumphs of the program was a pilot who had broken his back when he ditched his plane. After six months in plaster in hospital with no expectation of full recovery, he entered an air force convalescent hospital. Five weeks later he was able to perform seventy-five 'sit-ups' and return to normal duty.

Fliers' 'fatigue' was a similarly perplexing condition, but usually without an easily identified triggering event. It seemed to creep up on men. Again, air force convalescent hospitals developed a specialised treatment programme that they claimed could return men to normal duties months ahead of schedule. The technique consisted of an intensive application of vocational and physical activities in workshops, gymnasiums and on playing fields.

As a result, greatly increased numbers of otherwise 'useless' personnel were able to return to new duties, or new training, or be honourably discharged in reasonable health. The process was regarded as a form of human engineering that was not a perfect solution, but an improvement on most others. After all, it was just as necessary to prepare young men for civilian life as it was to prepare them to return to war. Armies in peacetime can review their medical experience with combat injuries and establish new procedures and rehabilitation techniques. The early management of severe head injuries is seen as a critical point in their care because attention to speech disorders, headache control, restoration of skull defects and suppression of post-traumatic epilepsy become critical later.

However, it was seen that little or no definitive neurosurgery could be performed in field hospitals as it required the specialised skills of evacuation hospitals with an inevitable delay of treatment during evacuation. The development of military neurosurgery had needed a big event like the Second World War to derive a large experience in management of penetrating head wounds. A single neurosurgical team could only treat half a dozen major head injuries in a twelve-hour session but, in 1944, army hospitals admitted 2,500 men for brain surgery – all requiring immediate, prolonged and expert rehabilitation for restoration of social, behavioural and speech deficits.

At the end of the Second World War, serious attention was directed for the first time to the question of how well Australian prisoners of the Japanese fared in civilian life after discharge from the forces. Nearly 2,000 veterans – half of them ex-prisoners – from the same theatres of war were traced for forty years. Dr Malcolm Dent and his psychiatric colleagues studied the impact of being a prisoner on men's post-war survival patterns. When their mortality was compared within the first fifteen years post-war, those who had been prisoners were somewhat more likely to have died than non-prisoners. As time passed, the difference was less obvious. Furthermore, younger men who had been imprisoned were found to be more likely to die early.

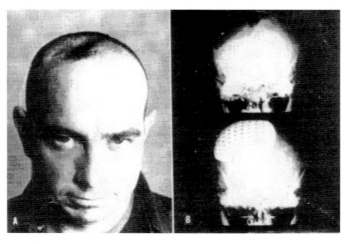

Healed depressed fracture of skull after scalp and bone shattering (left), treated later (right) by insertion of protective metal plate with in-growth holes seen at top left. (*US Army*)

We can summarise some of the great lessons of the Second World War by noting that it was fought over vast distances and with medical personnel of very variable experience, especially those of US and Australian forces spread across the Pacific where tropical diseases, including gas gangrene, were added to the military injuries of the drier climates of North Africa.

For the first and only time in history, atomic weapons were employed. The appointment of surgical 'consultants' as teachers, organisers and reporters of surgical competence and daily needs was a master stroke, as it had been in earlier wars. The staged management of injuries including shell-shock, rapid retrieval of the injured, triage, avoidance of cold injuries, the standardised treatment of contaminated wounds, full documentation of initial and staged procedures involving drainage and closure-timing, the place of antibiotics, transfusion and fracture-immobilisation have become fundamental tools that now have permanent places in all forms of surgical practice.

CHAPTER 13

Nuremberg and Other Agonies

Stop all the clocks, cut off the telephone.
Prevent the dog from barking with a juicy bone.
Silence the pianos and with muffled drum
Bring out the coffin, let the mourners come.
The stars are not wanted now: put out every one;
Pack up the moon and dismantle the sun;
Pour away the ocean and sweep up the wood;
For nothing now can ever come to any good.

– W. H. Auden, *Song IX, Funeral Blues*, 1936

The concentration of prisoners in camps with inadequate nutrition, sanitation and medical services can, of itself, produce epidemics that may serve the purpose of genocide. So-called 'concentration camps', such as those in Nazi Germany and in Stalin's 'gulag archipelago', had that as one of their intentions. These were not quarantine stations of foreign nationals, but places of systematic neglect and inevitable, active or passive extermination. Medical and psychiatric staff were certainly available, but no medical assistance was provided.

During the 1930s, Nazi Party congresses and rallies had frequently been held in Nuremberg, a small city in southern Germany. In the sixteenth century, it had been the centre of a German renaissance. Symbolically, Hitler staged huge propaganda events there in 1933 and later. In 1946 and 1947, Nuremberg became even more notorious as the location for trials of Nazi war criminals brought before international military tribunals.

In his opening statement in 1946, a prosecuting officer, Brigadier General Telford Taylor, remarked that:

A nation which deliberately infects itself with poison, will inevitably sicken and die. Germany was converted into an infernal combination of a lunatic asylum and a charnel house. The crimes were the result of sinister doctrines which sealed the fate of Germany, shattered Europe and left the world in ferment.

In examining the 'State Medical Services of the Third Reich', twenty-three defendant doctors were placed in the witness box, nineteen of whom had been in the medical services of the German state. Three were acquitted and twenty were found guilty of war crimes and crimes against humanity. One committed suicide before sentencing, and their leader, Karl Brandt, and eleven others were executed. Seven were imprisoned for periods of fifteen years to life. Their power had come directly from Hitler who directed the medical services of the German air force, army and, particularly, the SS troops of the Nazi Party. In 1942, Hitler had appointed Brandt, then aged thirty-two, as Supreme Medical Authority of the Reich. He headed the Office for Scientific and Medical Research with a 'Euthanasia Programme' to exterminate those of unsound body or mind. Brandt's medical credentials for such high command are unknown, but he had been an early member of the SS and was Hitler's personal 'escort physician'. A month before he was arrested by the British in May 1945, he had been condemned to death by a Berlin court for unspecified 'misdemeanours', but was released by the personal order of Admiral Doenitz.

Brandt's abrogation of every medical ethic involved the design and administration of concentration camps, the investigation of ethnic superiority and inferiority, and the conduct of living, human experimentation. Those so-called investigations included observations of people being frozen to death or killed by poisoned bullets, methods of euthanasia, the effects of submission to simulated high-altitude living without oxygen, aggravated cold, the intravenous infusion of seawater, carbolic acid and gasoline and the administration of mustard gas and phosphorus.

Cumulatively, the trial accounts make unbearable reading despite much of the language being, alternately, so highly scientific or unscientific as to obscure the awful clinical details. Records revealed how terrified individuals died in agony under the cold eyes of the physicians and scientists who designed the protocols and then observed and recorded minute details of the manner of death.

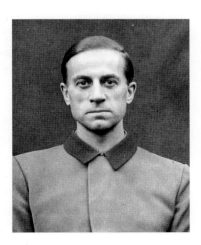

Dr Karl Brandt, Second World War Supreme
Medical Authority of Third Reich, aged thirty-two.
(*Heidi Epstein*)

The Nuremberg Principles, drafted in August 1945, now constitute the basis for all war crimes prosecutions; enquiries based on them were instituted in Yugoslavia in 1992 and in Rwanda in 2007. The concept of 'informed consent' was revisited in the 'Nuremberg Code' and further explored in the 'Helsinki Declaration' of 1964. They defined the general principles of involving human subjects in research, particularly in the context of a potential conflict of interest between the physician as a doctor and the physician as a researcher.

That issue was raised again in 2006 when Al-Jazeera News Network published shocking images of civilian casualties in an Iraq hospital. Questions were raised then about the ethics of both the media and hospital staff in showing that material. Many felt that the boundaries of decency and discretion had been severely tested by the needless and repeated use of gruesome footage.

The sinister objectives of the German procedures concerned: how to rescue or cure damaged and disabled humans, how to destroy or kill them if salvage failed, how to sterilise unwanted people, and how quickly various poisons work. The investigation of these macabre questions 'logically' involved the slaughter of 'enemies of the state' – Jews, Gypsies, Poles, Russians and the mentally defective. All investigations and procedures were highly planned and integrated by doctors, but none of their victims was a volunteer. Remarkably, the Nazi Party had passed rigid laws in 1933 for the protection of animals.

All doctors on trial had violated Hippocratic commandments on countless occasions and two of them came from senior posts in distinguished surgical departments. They had all agreed on certain Nazi principles:

> We would have to put to death, not only the mentally sick and the psychopathic personalities, but all the crippled, including the disabled veterans, old maids who do not work, all widows whose children had completed their education and all those living on their income or pensions.

At the end of a long year of evidence of depraved conduct, the Tribunal summarised the situation simply:

> This conspiracy was ... a ghastly failure as well as a hideous crime. The perpetrators showed neither courage nor wisdom nor vestiges of moral character.

The stories of Buchenwald, Pilsen and other camps have been told by soldiers, politicians, individuals and media. A doctor at war may see the situation in a somewhat more objective and analytical light than others but there was uniform revulsion felt by all who read or heard the evidence. Horrifying observations of concentration camps were made by James K. Sunshine at the end of his European war experience, and Colonel Elliott C. Cutler made the following notes after visiting Buchenwald in April 1945:

The original camp was built in 1937 for 7,000 people ... the camp had been used for political prisoners, not war prisoners originally. We were shown the crematorium with the beating room beneath it ... 30 or 40 patients who were taken out daily for an injection, died and never returned to the ward ... one ward housed children ... 3,400 inmates died. In the hospital ... in a laboratory tattooed sections of human skin, a pet hobby of the former commanding officer ... a total of 51,000 people died in this camp ... in the beating room beneath the crematorium there were hooks from the walls where men were strangled ... they had a noise machine so that the cries of the dying could not be heard elsewhere ... sometimes young people died ... an obvious starvation policy was evident ... many men breathing with difficulty ... and soon to die ... men with tuberculosis in bed together, coughing with each other ... the Germans of the nearby population felt no responsibility ... said they did not know it was going on (but) were turned out to watch hangings of prisoners ... 7,000 Russian soldiers were shot in the neck ... against a wall.

A similar trial of twenty-five Japanese doctors was held in Tokyo between May 1946 and November 1948, as a result of which seven were hanged, sixteen were imprisoned for life and two received long prison sentences. Never before had Japanese doctors been convicted en masse for crimes that ran counter to every ethic of the practice of medicine. The Nazi crimes such as murder, extermination, enslavement, persecution and bizarre experiments made no possible contribution to fundamental medical knowledge. Similar experiments had been conducted in northern China by the Japanese Germ Warfare Unit, accounting for the deaths of 10,000 Chinese and Allied prisoners.

In 2006, Dr Akira Makino of the Imperial Japanese Navy Medical Corps admitted to conducting vivisection on thirty prisoners of war in the Philippines during the Second World War. He described amputations, stitching of blood vessels and purposeless explorations of the abdominal cavity of 'subjects' until

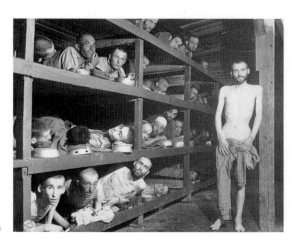

A 'Hospital ward' at Buchenwald Concentration Camp, Germany, Second World War. (*J. K. Sunshine*)

as late as 1945. At the end of his experiments, the captives were strangled. Dr Makino wanted to '... tell the truth about war to as many people as possible. If ... given the opportunity, I will continue to testify in atonement.' In fact, he had been lecturing high school students for years about his war experiences without once mentioning his human dissections.

By way of contrast, in September 2004 elderly residents of Arnhem gathered to honour the memory of a local surgeon. Sixty years earlier, he had been shot by the Nazis for helping injured British soldiers during fierce fighting in the Dutch city. In the Battle of Arnhem, nearly 4,000 British and Polish paratroopers had been killed or wounded. The residents met to install a plaque in the city centre, which read: 'In remembrance of Jaze Zwolle, doctor, shot 19 September 1944.'

The corruption of human dignity by doctors involved in interrogation of military prisoners was raised in 2006 with the deaths of three prisoners in the US prison at Guantanamo Bay, Cuba. While the nature of the doctors' involvement is not altogether clear, renewed vigilance was ordered to protect individuals from violations of human rights in such places.

In 2008–09, the US administration undertook a total review of the management of those who were incarcerated, with or without torture, for suspected terrorist activities. Investigation is ongoing.

CHAPTER 14

'Small' Wars

Frankly, I would like to see the government get out of war altogether and leave the whole field to private individuals.

– Joseph Heller, *Catch 22, 1961*

In the no-man's-lands of sub-Saharan Africa, streams of aeroplanes daily unload wounded civilians and combatants for surgical and medical care by teams of foreign and indigenous surgeons. Ninety per cent of victims are civilians, with one third of them children who have been maimed or killed by mines, bullets or cluster bombs as in Cambodia, Iraq, Nicaragua, Afghanistan, Palestine, Sierra and Sri Lanka. In fact, none of the third world is free from continuous conflict. It is an absurd reality that so many of the most deprived nations on earth are simultaneously being plundered of their enormous natural wealth by affluent, marauding multinationals. One member of a recent American humanitarian mission had worked at the rambling JFK Hospital in Monrovia, Liberia. He went home saying:

> The children of these countries are our children. We would never have believed that surgery could be carried out in such conditions. When today someone goes to war, the correct translation of that war is slaughter of civilians nine times out of ten. Wars do not end with peace treaties. Land mines have a life span of several decades, continuing to maim people years after they have been planted in the ground. 350 models of anti-personnel mines are manufactured by American, Chinese, Italian and Russian companies. They create an army of mutilated children. These devices are designed to maim people, not kill them. As a result, the contexts of war have changed and they have become endless wars.

Hospital records in Kabul, Afghanistan, show that most of the war injured are also non-combatants – children, females and the elderly. But the damage doesn't stop with effective surgery. There is an impossibly large need for burns units, rehabilitation centres, orthopaedic and physiotherapy departments and immense numbers of prosthetic devices. Most of the injured will never receive an artificial limb. If children are lucky enough to receive one, they are unlikely to ever get a replacement as their bodies grow.

Humanitarian organisations such as the International Red Cross (IRC) and Médecins Sans Frontières (MSF) produce a vast number of educational materials for the teaching of modern techniques to the populations of neglected areas. The complexity of these needs in 'small' modern wars is reflected in a list of topics and programmes made constantly available to indigenous surgeons, nurses and civilians. It is a very pragmatic list and few of us would foresee all these needs:

Management of dead bodies, intended for use by those first on the scene following a disaster when no specialists are at hand; teaching the recovery, identification, storage and disposal of the dead.

Water sanitation, hygiene and habitat in prisons.

Hospitals for the war-wounded: a practical guide for setting up and running a surgical hospital in an area of armed conflict with unprecedented influxes of casualties.

Manuals of nutrition.

War wounds: management of effects of missiles or explosions.

Amputations in war.

Caring for landmine victims, those disabled for life and needing long term care, not only rehabilitation but social and economic support.

Physical rehabilitation programs.

First aid and means of triage.

Skin grafting.

Treatment of infections.

Plastic surgery.

Anaesthesia.

Techniques of rapid amputation for victims of anti-personnel mines and other explosive devices.

It may come as a surprise that, in 2007, the Australian Department of Foreign Affairs and Trade advised against all non-vital travel to most of the central African states, Iraq and Afghanistan, and strongly warned against travel to some northern African states, parts of South America, East Timor, Haiti, Indonesia, Israel, Lebanon, Pakistan, Saudi Arabia, Sri Lanka and Syria. Savage insurgents and marauders wish it to stay that way.

However, doctors and nurses of humanitarian groups ignore the risks, even when they may be attacked or kidnapped for having suspected political intent. They can also be injured by stray bullets or mines, or affected by the same epidemics that they are treating. Frequently, medical teams are urgently evacuated because of excessive war risks to their lives.

We live in an age of guerrilla and terrorist warfare. Battlefronts are smaller and more commonly in civilian areas. The wounds of hand-to-hand combat are diminishing in most of the world, apart from the unrelenting conflicts of

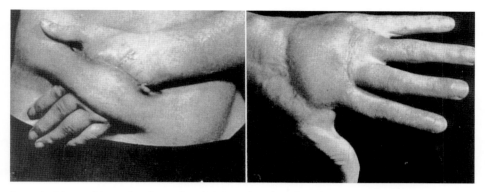

Staged skin-grafting of a large hand injury by skin flap from patient's abdomen. Left shows flap initially attached to the abdomen for wound coverage and, at right, the flap is separated and tailored to freely cover the hand defect. The abdominal wound will be grafted later. (*US Army*)

Africa and the Third World. The trench warfare of the First World War will not be seen again. Even the poorest nations' militias and children may be armed with automatic weapons, grenades, mines and bombs. The devastating effects of remotely controlled explosive devises are increasingly evident. Every day, terrorists kill themselves for no conventional military or religious reasons and produce multiple and unpredictable injuries to civilian and military targets alike. Their aim is terrorise their enemies – even if that means hurting innocent bystanders – and the result places maximum demands on surgical and medical resources in varying locations.

In modern wars, surgery is nothing like civilian trauma surgery. It differs because of the nature of injuries, the number of casualties occurring simultaneously, the number of malnourished and diseased patients, the austerity of surgical workplaces and the limited numbers of diagnostic resources and speciality consultants. Surgeons in the field must be prepared to quickly deal with many massive wounds, logistical breakdown, hostile fire, limited evacuation of the wounded and the overwhelming confusion of all wars.

Civilians and most medical people find triage an intuitively repellent concept, but the general aims and principles of military surgery remain as they always were – to fix what you can and to avoid futile treatment for those you cannot help. The first military priority of all care for the injured is to maintain operational capability. That is done by returning as many soldiers as possible to combat as quickly as possible.

A recent president of the American College of Surgeons, Dr Kathryn Anderson, described surgery as '… the greatest humanitarian profession in the world' and that is undoubtedly true. It is also inevitable that early and better surgical management has produced such remarkable survival that rehabilitation needs have far exceeded those presently available anywhere, especially in poor countries. Clearly, the same has become apparent in American military rehabilitation hospitals of today.

VIETNAM

The Vietnam War originated in the threat of communist domination of the region, where booby traps and small arms injuries resulted in the admission of 150,000 Americans to army hospitals between 1965 and 1971. Luckily, badly wounded men could often reach definitive care within ninety minutes of injury.

Although one in every forty of them died, it was still only half the rate of dying that occurred in the Second World War. In every war since then, the mortality rate from serious wounding has diminished, largely because of speedier evacuation, expert treatment of shock and the use of urgent, expert surgical repair. About 50,000 Australian troops served alongside 200,000 Americans in Vietnam from 1965 onward. Five per cent of the diggers had major wounds and 1 per cent died.

As was experienced in 'big' wars, most mortality was related directly to a state of shock in which a reduction of effective blood volume led to a fall in blood pressure in critical tissues. The result was progressive and permanent failure of body organs. If the worst of the injured were to survive, transfusion had to be early and copious. If that was to be possible, the army needed helicopters able to fly at night and pressurised aircraft for high-altitude transportation.

An alarming and original autopsy finding in many young Americans who died in Vietnam was significant degenerative pathology in their coronary and cerebral arteries. Many non-combat deaths were attributed specifically to such a disease. Medical staff in Vietnam noted unusual symptoms in a number of 'disturbed' men – during and after their service. It was often impossible to confidently explain complaints from men who showed no physical injury or other conventional abnormality. Others exhibited a syndrome not quite like the 'shell-shock' of the First and Second World Wars. Many doctors found diversionary influences difficult to separate from the effects of the environment of war, particularly when many troops used unquantifiable doses of recreational drugs.

Some carers theorised that the strange symptoms may have been the result of troops' recent experiences in civilian life. They often came from a background of the 'psychedelic counter-culture' common in those years, involving disturbing religions, flower-power, hippy-living, hallucinogens, concepts of mind-control and widespread, experimental social-engineering.

Whatever the impact of that was on how troops and their medical attendants responded, morale was further disturbed by a constant barrage of criticism of the war from civilians in the United States and many other countries. They saw many barbaric incidents such as the infamous image of a Viet Cong suspect being shot through the head by a Vietnamese general.

One correspondent estimated that, on that single night, the shooting was witnessed by 25 million people on TV. By contrast, polls showed that most of those watching the 'routine' American evening TV news had no recollection next day of the specific issues which the anchorman had reported, but they clearly recalled the abhorrent picture.

It is not altogether surprising that there was a common view, shared by some senior North Vietnamese Army officers, that the media, particularly TV, had finally lost the war for the United States. If there were any doubts about that, there were even fewer after the repeated showing of an American soldier incinerating a Vietnamese hut with a cigarette lighter, even though it was suggested later that the incident had been staged for the cameras.

Another disturbing ingredient in the twelve years of that war was the media coverage of varied events, showing that the most terrible things were always happening somewhere in the world. One had only to look at the Civil Rights Movement, the Afro-American Rights conflict in the American South, the Detroit and Newark riots, the assassination of Martin Luther King, the Bay of Pigs crisis in Cuba, the assassinations of John and Robert Kennedy and the Six Days War in the Middle East.

Inevitably, that sort of material increasingly filled and confused men's minds until they turned to their doctors for help with baffling symptoms. It is easy to forget that medical teams were at least as influenced by the issues as the men they treated – sometimes more so. They suffered frustration at persisting difficulties in reconciling physical and functional complaints and their complete inability to assist recovery. They were not immune to such themes, but how could they be?

Some of them may also have experienced a response that some psychiatrists termed 'catastrophisation' – a variant form of panic disorder where a subject may have difficulty in isolating particular from multiple issues and have distorted value systems. That made it impossible to discriminate the good from the bad, or even fact from fiction. Clearly, that could seriously reduce a soldier's combat competence or a surgeon's efficiency in an operative situation.

American troops and medical teams were found to be affected by a strong, isolationist, anti-draft movement made up of those who were unwilling to be enlisted for war. On student campuses there was growing dissent on a whole range of matters put forward by highly-publicised, conscientious objectors. No wonder that America finally accepted the wisdom of pulling its military and medical teams out of Vietnam.

It is no surprise that conditions experienced by a foot-soldier in Vietnam were very different from those of senior commanders and medical staff. A senior Australian surgeon, Dr Gordon Ormandy, described his surgical service in Vietnam as little worse than his long experience of violent trauma in a large, industrial city in Australia. Similarly, Dr Marshall Barr, a specialist anaesthetist with the Australian Army in Vietnam, described a very varied experience with periods of relative idleness and recreation alternating with periods of intense repulsion from the ugliness of massive injuries.

Barr's description of his recreational activities is illuminating:

> [They were] ... the envy of any combat soldier at Nui Dat or those drearily trapped in the logistic support group ... rewarding work without any great danger ... opportunities to play and ... see something of the country ... a brief and molly-coddled tour.

That description seems an understatement from a doctor who also described, with great sensitivity and frankness, some of the worst elements of his war:

> ... the crushing overload of work from the Tet offensive ... more than I realised ... it took months to get back to some sort of normality ... the stress of the fearful responsibility had got to [other medical staff] ... I had totally failed to appreciate the emotional trauma being inflicted on our young medics ... doctors and nurses become hardened by training and experience

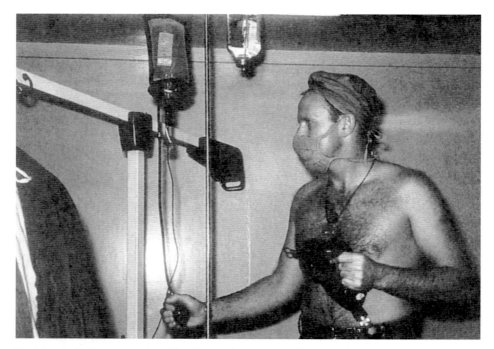

Dr Marshall Barr pumping blood transfusion with his right hand and ventilating the patient's lungs with his left hand, Vietnam, 1968. (*Allen & Unwin P/L*)

and have a controlled process of gradual exposure ... to Australia's appalling toll of road trauma ... dealing with shattered young bodies ... operating theatre technicians had no comparable background ... they responded so professionally to our training and performed so well when the casualties began to arrive, that I accepted their apparent calmness without question.

During more than twenty years of war, 100,000 Vietnamese people lost limbs, with many more in Cambodia and Laos – casualties keep occurring even today. Rehabilitation of those casualties and others with war wounds, as well as civilian injuries, required eight major, full-time Red Cross rehabilitation centres and sixty offices. They continue to freely distribute care, advice, training and medical services – perhaps to continue forever – at little or no cost to those countries.

KOREA

Between 1950 and 1953, when communist North Korean forces, supported by Russia and China, invaded the south, 40,000 Americans and 2½ million Koreans and Chinese people died. Countless civilian casualties on both sides were displaced or slaughtered before an uneasy détente was forged. The supreme priority of quickly moving the injured to places of expert care became

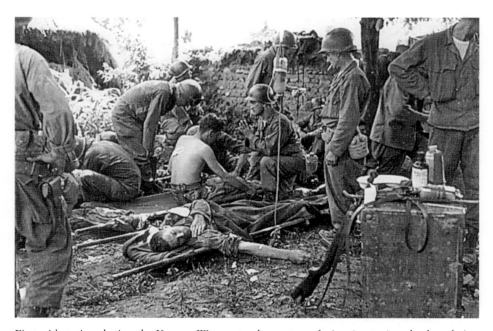

First-aid station during the Korean War; note plasma transfusion (centre) and others being treated by medics. (*US Army*)

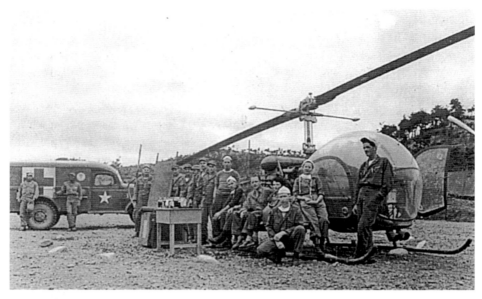

A helicopter rescue crew with pilots, nurses, medics and mechanics; first used extensively in Korea. (*US Army*)

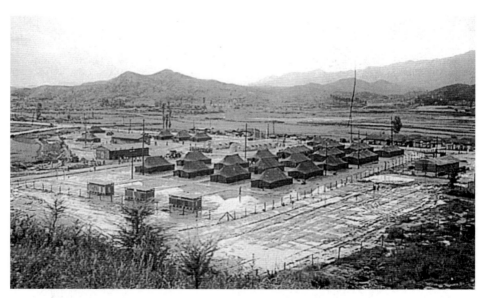

Mobile surgical hospital, Korea, 1951; living quarters, hospital wards and an airfield are seen beyond beyond. (*US Army*)

obvious as never before. Helicopters and 'MASH' units were often providing definitive treatment within six hours of a man being wounded. The repair of blood-vessels in limbs lowered clean amputation rates from 50 per cent to 15 per cent. Battlefield kidney dialysis became a new possibility for salvaging the deeply shocked patient, even in forward areas.

Never before had such complex medical activity been possible, assisted by the availability of penicillin that made it feasible to perform the worst forms of complex abdominal surgery with reasonable salvage rates. Despite the prolonged confusion, civilian loss and disruption of the war, South Korea is today a flourishing state with advanced surgical services. Meanwhile, the primary aggressor, North Korea, remains economically stressed and poorly advanced.

IRAQ'S DESERT STORM

Medical commanders in Iraq's 1990 'Desert Storm' operation soon discovered that, just as the 'great' wars had shown their predecessors, the most recently enlisted army doctors were not experienced in caring for severe injuries. Few of them had ever worked in metropolitan emergency rooms and even fewer

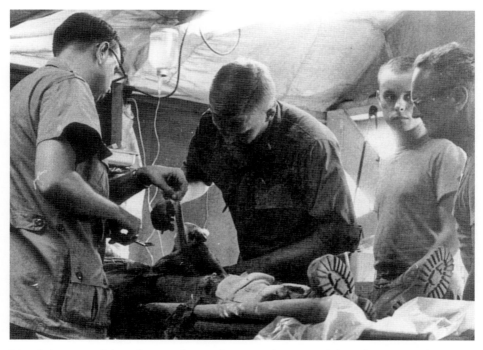

Man being treated for a haemorrhaging leg wound in Iraq while still on a stretcher in his boots, with plasma transfusion running. (*Dr G. Peoples*)

had treated bullet and shrapnel wounds. As it transpired, Coalition casualties were few and the results of surgery remarkable, particularly when treatment was carried out in ideal circumstances on board USNS *Comfort*, a 1,000-bed hospital ship located close offshore and staffed by more than fifty specialist surgical teams. They had the great advantage that wounded men were otherwise healthy, vaccinated and immunised. In addition, they were freshly evacuated, and there was plenty of blood and antibiotics. The result was a much higher yield of survival than in any previous war.

BOUGAINVILLE

During the Bougainville civil war between 1997 and 2003, locals were seeking political independence from Papua New Guinea. Because of the fighting, a great deal of surgery was required for civilians. One in every four of those treated by Australian and New Zealand surgical services was a child. It was one of the first times in reported war that teams were parachuted in to set up and operate surgical facilities. The same techniques were applied by the same services in East Timor's protracted wars of independence.

The skills required for work in remote areas cannot exist adequately in any single surgeon, simply because of the extremely unpredictable combat surgery required and the unusually complex forms of civilian pathology encountered. Military surgeons in such places need personal and group expertise across a wide range of procedures, including paediatrics and obstetrics.

With increasing experience, severe abdominal injuries that were once a death sentence from uncontrollable haemorrhage and contamination by ruptured bowel became manageable, with a halving of mortality rates. Newer techniques involved bowel decompression and partial closure of the abdomen cavity until the patient's condition had stabilised enough to allow evacuation to specialist centres. Similar principles had been described originally by Dr Michael E. DeBakey and his colleagues in the Second World War.

ISRAEL AND LEBANON

At a recent surgical conference in the Middle East following the Hezbollah–Israeli conflict of July 2006, it was reported that a 350-bed Israeli hospital had been hit by a rocket, wounding eight people including a surgeon. Other Israeli hospitals admitted more than 400 citizens wounded by Hezbollah rockets fired from up to 100 kilometres away. Two hundred rockets had been sent daily, resulting in seventeen Israeli deaths and 1,500 injured. Many required intensive treatment for anxiety. From the other side of that combat, Lebanese medical staff reported that Israeli aircraft destroyed two Red Cross ambulances bringing wounded civilians to hospital, seriously injuring six Red Cross medical staff and three patients. Both ambulances had been clearly marked by flashing lights, sirens and Red Cross symbols. Clearly, there are no effective rules of war and the same accusations persist wherever it is happening.

HAITI

Working with other organisations such as the Red Cross, the Sisters of Charity of Calcutta and the Brothers of Bangladesh, MSF has tried to deal with the recurrent waves of violence witnessed in the civil war in Haiti, which continues despite the presence of UN peacekeeping forces and a partial transition to a form of democracy. Women and children are shot indiscriminately, often in the back, as they flee from violence. Specialist visiting surgeons assisting the native medical staff have expereienced great difficulties from a lack of even the simplest hardware. At one hospital, they found none of six lung ventilators and only four of six operating tables in working order. Ambulances and sterilising equipment hadn't been in service for five years. There was no waste treatment and a power generator was defective, but the visitors stayed until they were forced to leave by threats to their lives.

An MSF nurse in Haiti told of 5,000 patients treated in one hospital in a year – half of them for gunshot wounds and other violence. Half were women, children or elderly. There was an everlasting shortage of blood for transfusion.

On one day there were twenty-eight emergency operations for wounds by fragmentation bullets that smashed soft tissues and bones to pieces. After dusk, staff were in danger both in the hospital and if they attempted to leave for home, simply because too few security men were in the hospitals or on the streets to protect them from the crossfire of crazed marauding militias.

As if Haiti's agonies were not already intolerable, its strongest earthquake in 200 years struck in January 2010, followed by a crushing tsunami. The resulting chaos and desolation will require massive reconstruction with enormous help provided by the wider world. Haiti's medical and surgical services may ultimately benefit from such an infusion of expertise, equipment, rebuilding and internal discipline.

CONGO BASIN

One American surgeon working in the resource-rich Congo has spent the whole of her recent surgical life operating on victims of a civil war. That involves adults and children with gunshot and machete wounds, burns and injuries of gross sexual violence. She had previously done the same in Sri Lanka and

Burundi. Her team manages up to forty surgical cases each day, many times more than would ever be performed in the United States.

On one day the surgeon treated young children who had been seriously wounded by guns and knives and a teenage girl who had been shot four times. Two teenage girls had been repeatedly raped, causing severe pelvic damage, and another was moribund after being held by four men who raped her every day for a month. Between 2003 and 2005, MSF treated 2,500 victims of sexual violence in men, women and children of all ages. Most surgery in the Congo is directed towards trying to save injured limbs from infections that would make amputation essential. Whatever the stresses of performing surgery, volunteers have learned to not express their opinions in local politics. To 'take-sides' by word or action merely compounds medical difficulties and invites death to patients and staff alike.

Lately, Rwanda has become implicated in a more violent civil war originating in East Congo between various guerrilla factions responsible for killing and disabling thousands of innocent civilians. Since 2008, the numbers of victims have greatly increased despite a UN-assisted intervention to eradicate Rwandan rebels with the help of the Congolese and Rwandan armies.

Such has been the level of constant danger that medical services can no longer be maintained by humanitarian agencies.

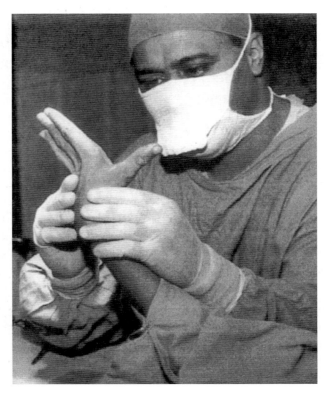

A military surgeon treating the deformed hand of a civilian, Congo, 2003. (*IRC*)

SUDAN

For some twenty-five years a civil war over political dominance has been continuing in the state of Darfur in western Sudan. The victims of the fighting have been served by many itinerant Red Cross surgical teams who set up mobile Field Surgical Hospitals. Staffed by one surgeon, one anaesthetist and two nurses, their work is endangered by being in zones of constant armed conflict between warring parties accused of genocide and ethnic cleansing. The common sequence following the violence is displacement of villagers that produces starvation and illnesses that kill thousands.

The Red Cross groups attend to any civilian or combatant beyond the reach of surgical care in hospital, but do not work in active combat areas. The most common surgical services – usually carried out in improvised surgical facilities – are for rapes, fractures, chest and abdominal injuries, and burns. Many of their patients arrive in trucks and cars that have travelled great distances from areas of war. In a typical day in this dangerous environment, where poor transportation limits numbers, the Red Cross teams still work for up to twenty hours non-stop and perform twenty-five to thirty operations per visit. Then they leave to do the same elsewhere on the next and every other day.

Ever since an 'official' peace was declared in 2005, southern Sudan has sustained hundreds of dead and thousands of injured from a civil war which

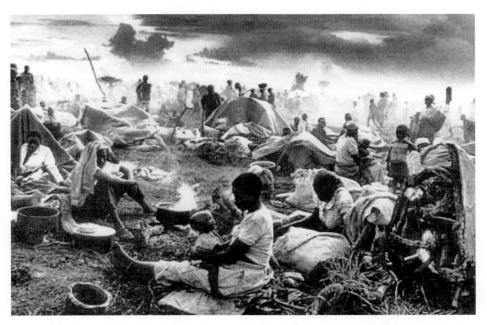

The chaos of a third world refugee camp, probably Darfur, with no medical care in sight. (*International Red Cross (IRC)*)

escalated steeply in 2009. Rebel groups in Uganda and the Democratic Republic of the Congo (DRC) have forced thousands of Sudanese to flee across the borders of adjacent states. Medical help is no longer available to these refugees. Similarly, in Darfur, millions of displaced people have been threatened by the Sudanese government's eviction of international agencies from the country since its President's indictment on charges of war crimes.

KENYA

Lopiding Red Cross Hospital in Lokichokio is the largest field hospital in the world. It was established in 1987 to care for 700 patients, mostly airlifted victims of conflict in southern Sudan. Its surgeons perform 5,000 operations yearly, many for multiple injuries, in two operating theatres with some intensive care and support services. Its orthopaedic workshop has fitted 5,000 artificial limbs and dispensed 10,000 pairs of crutches.

Loki airport accommodates British, American and Russian Medevac transport planes flying a 'milk-run' service to ferry patients to and from Sudan and settlements scattered around the Nile. While most patients were once the war-wounded, today they are more often the casualties of 'peace' – of violent civil unrest, complicated diseases and infections, trauma and snakebites. In twenty years of war, 2 million Sudanese have died and millions have been displaced from their homes.

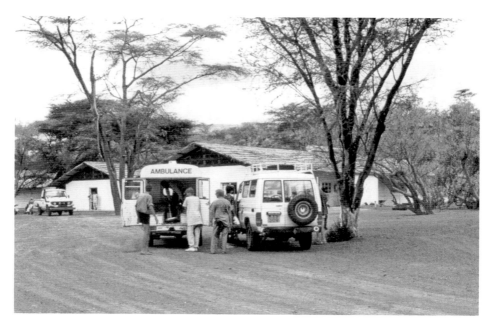

Ambulances at Lopiding Red Cross Hospital, Kenya, 1987. (*IRC*)

SOMALIA

Despite a presidential change and UN assistance, the combination of severe drought, unremitting violence and the systematic aggression against aid workers has caused Somalia to lose all national and humanitarian health aid in the last year. In and around the capital Mogadishu, emergency surgical assistance has been attempted intermittently, but fighting between government and rebel forces has resulted in huge loss of life, starvation and the displacement of millions.

The stereotyped pattern of these wars follows predictable steps – indiscriminate killing and wounding, starvation, displacement of civilians from their homes and rejection of all offers of health-care. It is difficult to foresee improvements in such elemental defects of management.

RWANDA

The unrelenting civil war between extreme ethnic groups trying to enforce domination by extreme methods of genocide is characteristic of much of African violence today. It is worsened by resource plundering, regardless of the presence of UN and other peacekeepers. In 1994 alone, more than a million civilians were slaughtered or rendered homeless in Rwanda – an impossible task for humanitarian medical teams to confront effectively.

PAKISTAN

Conflict between the army and heavily-armed opposition groups was exacerbated during 2009 by bombing of large cities, including hospitals and health clinics, causing thousands of deaths, injuries and 2 million displaced civilians. Among the deaths were two MSF workers whose cross-marked ambulance was attacked while evacuating injured townspeople. Other doctors and nurses were similarly attacked. By May 2009, over a million civilians had been so threatened by ground warfare and bombing that they had fled into conditions of isolation, famine and drought.

SRI LANKA

After decades of conflict between government forces and the revolutionary Tamil Tigers in the north-east, many thousands of anti-government civilians became isolated to a narrow coastal strip where there was no protection and little food or medical care.

Since the government expelled most aid agencies, IRC workers have attempted to continue care of critically ill civilians. They have assisted in the evacuation of many of those threatened, but by mid-2009 thousands suffering from malnutrition, gunshot, shrapnel and land-mine injuries without adequate medical care had been incarcerated in makeshift northern camps where it was difficult to maintain surgical units. In the last quarter of 2009, many civilians were allowed to leave the camps and untold numbers have fled Sri Lanka to seek asylum overseas.

NORTHERN YEMEN

The year 2009 saw the worst of the country's long history of violence when the army sought to suppress Al-Houti rebels in a conflict that involved civilians and military targets in unprecedented numbers. Humanitarian assistance from MSF and other independent organisations was halted and hundreds of thousands were displaced. Established surgical teams were evacuated urgently with no plans to resume their work. Malnutrition and deficiency illnesses in children and adults of all ages was rife and the uninvited involvement of Saudi Arabian forces aggravated their deprivation more than they helped. At year's end, almost every state was affected by a raging conflict which defied all assistance.

CHAPTER 15

Iraq and Afghanistan

The first thing our guys are told is 'don't get captured'. They know they
will be tortured and beheaded [and shown] on the internet. Zarqawi [now
dead] openly offered bounties to anyone who brought him a live American
serviceman. This motivated the criminal elements who otherwise don't give a
hoot about the war. A lot of the beheading victims were actually kidnapped
by common criminals and sold to Zarqawi. As such, for our guys, every fight
is to the death. Surrender is not an option.

– US Marine, quoted by Robin Hardy, Iraq 2005

On 25 July 2006, Australian ABC Radio presented an interview with an
un-named doctor in Baghdad. His nationality, area of expertise, hospital
appointment and surgical experience were not revealed but there is no reason
to doubt his claims. There have been similar reports elsewhere:

Gunmen sometimes burst into operating theatres, shouting demands. If
you lose the patient, you pay by your life. Their friends should be treated
first; their enemies should be left to die – very much a breach of the code of
conduct of the medical system.

Another Iraqi doctor recently told Australian ABC Radio that crimes and
kidnapping against health workers are endemic in Iraq and little is known of
their fate. About 250 Iraqi doctors have catalogued human rights violations
including bombing and military raids on hospitals. Insurgent patients were
killed in their beds and ambulance transport of wounded combatants during
the siege of Fallujah was obstructed. Scores of surgeons reported harassment
and some were arrested on a pretext while actually performing operations.

A 2007 'Foreign Correspondent' report on ABC-TV, Sydney, featured Dr Al
Sheibani, an Iraqi surgeon working in the emergency and operating rooms of a
local Baghdad hospital, as he had done for the past fourteen years. Every week
his work involved caring for hundreds of Shiite civilians injured and dying
when caught in sectarian warfare and from improvised explosive devices and
suicide bombers. Blood and medical supplies were in short supply and nobody
could tell where the funds to provide them had gone. Operating conditions

were basic with no skilled assistants or refined surgical equipment, and there was no X-ray or ultrasound available.

Dr Al Sheibani's emergency rooms were crowded with uninjured civilians who impeded the activities of medical staff. Aggressive relatives and friends often filled ambulances carrying one slightly injured person. One fit-looking patient kept calling, 'We are strong mentally. God is great!'

Up to forty small operations were performed every day, but there was no security in the hospital. Surgical staff were told to obey orders from outsiders or be killed. The surgeon feared that Iraq would become a 'disaster zone' if the Americans and their allies left. He knew he was placing himself at risk by filming and discussing hospital conditions with the media. In fact, as the film ended, he was packing his bags to escape with his family before repercussions could eventuate.

Dr Al Sheibani and his colleagues believe that a majority of civilians could be saved if trained and experienced Iraqi staff are available – citing the typical ambulance that is manned only by a driver with no medical training. They deplore the lack of indigenous emergency facilities in Iraq. Its population of over 26 million has only 180 hospitals with few emergency departments and most 'acute' victims cannot be competently treated because their doctors have neither experience nor equipment. Worst of all, as members of an elite group in Iraq, doctors have become the targets of daily insurgent resentment. Many have been killed or kidnapped for ransom and others have fled the country or closed their clinics. Even if they know the criminals, nobody will say exactly who they are or their reasoning. Some doctors believe that poor-quality emergency services may be worse than leaving people untreated. There is a fear that services will decline further as Allied medical and surgical services are withdrawn progressively.

Karin Brulliard of *The Washington Post* reported that Iraqi health authorities were urgently trying to stem the large exodus of their doctors from the country. The government is refusing to issue diplomas to new graduates until they have completed at least six years in Iraqi hospitals, including experience with combat injuries. Officials are desperate to limit the doctors' expatriation to nearby Jordan and Syria and are offering incentives to stay at home. They include the provision of individual private clinics in public hospitals, subsidised accommodation and tight security to reduce attacks on doctors and their families.

Other reports confirm that the Ministry of Health had actually obstructed access of injured Iraqi troops and police to Iraqi hospitals. Why, nobody seems to know, but sectional politics, poor facilities and a bias against treating soldiers in civilian hospitals have been offered as contributing reasons for that attitude. Fortunately, most of the Iraqi wounded soldiers and civilians are still treated by doctors in American field hospitals. That luxury will be withdrawn progressively as the US winds down its commitment in Iraq.

BALAD

The brilliant concept of MASH units (Mobile Army Surgical Hospitals), attributed to Dr Michael E. DeBakey and others, originated in Italy at the end of the Second World War. They were used extensively in the Korean and Vietnam Wars and are employed in Iraq and Afghanistan today. The biggest military hospital in the world is at Balad, north of Baghdad, where the wounded are taken directly from MASH units in battle zones. If they arrive alive, 96 per cent of them will survive. In April 2006, an observer wrote:

> The constellation of injuries is unlike anything we have seen. Every once in a while a patient will have what we call a 'Balad special', which means we will have three or four surgical teams operating simultaneously [on the same patient] ... we all have to cooperate with each other and stay out of each other's way.

Staff Sergeant Jim Goodwin described a typical scene:

> As Marines [were] stamping out remaining pockets of insurgents in Fallujah ... in the first six days of the offensive, the 63 surgeons, nurses, corpsmen and other personnel of the Surgical Shock Trauma Platoon (SSTP) treated 157 patients, including 29 Iraqis, and performed 73 operations.

'We do damage-controlling, death-cheating surgery here' is how one operating room nurse in Balad referred to first aid, controlling haemorrhage, stabilising patients and preparing them for movement by aircraft to further treatment in even larger medical facilities overseas, such as in Germany and Spain.

One SSTP had so many casualties arriving by taxi-like ambulances that the road was blocked for hundreds of metres. Most of the men survived, due largely to the modern body-armour issued to Marines and the rapid, expert surgical care they got. 'If they weren't wearing their flak [vest] and Kevlar [helmet] they'd all have these [pointing to their heads and chests] damaged,' the nurse said. The survival rate of troops in Iraq now is almost twice that of Vietnam thirty years ago.

Cal Perry of *CNN* described a typical operating-room conversation in Balad:

> "Don't let me die! Please, don't let me die", an American soldier pleads as medics carry him to a trauma room. He sees an army chaplain kneeling over him. There is blood everywhere. A roadside bomb exploded next to his patrol vehicle, sending lumps of metal into his body and hurling him from the vehicle.
>
> "Am I going to live?" he asks over and over.

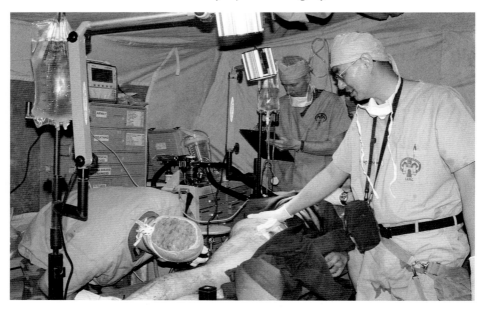

Surgeons assessing a patient before surgery with an anaesthetist in the background, Balad, 2004. (*Dr H. Stinger*)

"Hell, yes, you are," one of the doctors replies yet again.

The blast had torn soft tissue off his leg and his left hand was almost severed. Just breathe nice and deep, a surgeon told the soldier as his anaesthetic began.

"I'm not going to die, am I?"

"Don't you dare. I didn't give you permission."

"Am I going to lose the f……. leg?"

"I don't know. We'll save it if we can. OK? I just don't know."

The soldier kept his arm and leg but in the hallway, his buddy lay in a black bag.

Down the hall, the soldier who was driving the vehicle was better off than his buddies despite burnt hands and shrapnel in his neck: "It just exploded … on the left side or under the vehicle – I'm not sure – everything was on fire. I got out through the gunner's hatch and got one more out."

Another injured soldier called his wife in the US to explain what had happened to him: "I'm fine … you just go and pray."

Medics comment on what army surgeons do and see:

[Conditions that] … no doctors in the world have seen elsewhere – things that doctors in civilian life don't see, such as blast wounds, soldiers with their limbs blown off. The doctors are faced with emotional challenges that no other doctor is faced with. A soldier dies [while] doctors are saving another soldier's life. As doctors are pronouncing a soldier dead, they have to treat another soldier and save his life. They do it seven days a week, every day of the year because they have to. They treat insurgents too. It takes a toll on the doctors. But every day they have to face up to the war. They see it up close as it arrives. They will go home to save lives from car crashes. They will give it everything they have. To be able to cope with this and move onto the next day is something incredible.

David Zucchino reported in the *Los Angeles Times* about, 'Bringing back the wounded with heart, soul and surgery':

[The sergeant] ... lay shivering in a trauma bay. He felt something in his mouth. He sat up and spat fragments of his front teeth into a bedpan. They were mixed with blood and tissue from inside his mouth. He heard someone say "significant laceration of the cheek and lip, frag[ment] under the eye ... frag in the face ... frag in the shoulder ... possible thumb fractures".

A bomb fashioned from two mortar rounds had exploded behind him on patrol. He asked a doctor if he would need his face reconstructed and was told, "Nope, just some new teeth."

"My wife's going to be pissed off," he told the doctor. "She specifically gave me instructions not to get perforated over here." The sergeant looked down and saw a Purple Heart on his lap.

It was estimated that about 100 American troops were wounded in action in a typical week in Iraq in 2004. Massive bleeding was a major cause of death, but it is less common today due to an accelerated evacuation procedure to remove the wounded from the battlefield into an assembly line – first to emergency surgery and perhaps later to military hospitals in Europe and the USA. Helicopters can get them to a forward hospital within an hour of injury, but it is a long and hazardous hour.

During the Vietnam War, the nearest combat-support hospital was in Japan from which it took more than a month to evacuate a wounded soldier to a major US mainland hospital. In Iraq, the same sort of transfer now takes less than a week. Since the Iraq war began, about 10 per cent of wounded troops have died from their injuries – half at the point of injury and a half during surgery. The figures were 30 per cent during the Second World War and 24 per cent during the Vietnam War. One soldier in Balad had been wounded in combat nine months earlier and was back on duty in Iraq for two months before he was re-injured by an IED (Improvised Explosive Device). Again, he survived because of expert, ultra-rapid surgery.

Ballistic goggles, many of a more fashionable commercial design than standard issue, have saved the eyesight of thousands of men and body-

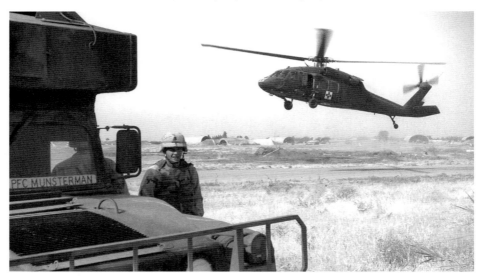

The evacuation of wounded men by a Black Hawk helicopter, Iraq. A medic in a Kevlar vest is in the foreground and a camp is in the distance. (*Dr G. Peoples*)

armour has saved the lives of many more. But faces, limbs, necks and armpits are still too exposed to damage and improved armour design is an urgent need.

Some of the wounded have described a strange sort of 'mental space' after injury when time stops and they wonder what has happened. It is as if they are watching somebody else. Others feel foolish and incompetent for getting hurt. They have to adjust to that attitude and counselling is immediately available, but it will take time to know how much it has helped. The amputation rate in Iraq, most as a result of IEDs, has been twice that of previous wars and many soldiers face the rest of their lives with severe eye or brain damage.

The most disturbing rescue missions of all involve the 'dead angels' – men who have been killed in action. Whenever possible, and as gently as if they were alive, their bodies are transported in dedicated vehicles. Far too many casualties arrive for surgical care in a category described by the accompanying medic as 'FUBAR' – military slang for 'Fouled Up Beyond All Repair' – doomed to die because they are in the 'hopeless' triage category.

One in that group was urgently brought into the trauma room unconscious – shocked and bleeding torrentially from somewhere inside his belly. A roadside bomb had lacerated his spleen, which had already been removed at an aid station. They stitched his bowel together there and packed his abdominal cavity to control internal bleeding from a hundred broken blood vessels and a torn liver. The surgical staff at Balad knew at once that he was near death with his blood pressure low, his tissues filled with acid and his kidneys failing. Somebody asked nobody in particular, 'What else can we do but try? He just

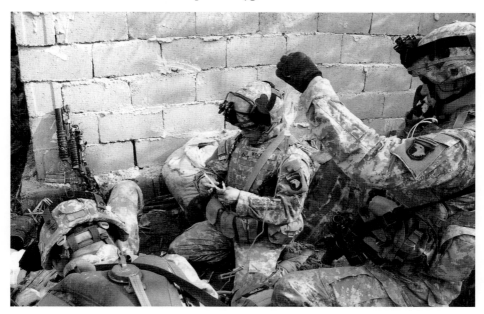

Urgent resuscitation by three medics in a battle area; the man in the centre is preparing syringes while the man on the right is giving plasma. All are in Kevlar, goggles and helmets. (*Dr H. Stinger*)

might get to cross an ocean to home again, mightn't he?' Nobody answered and he died within an hour.

Three or more helicopters and crews are constantly on call, waiting to transport the injured to Balad with medics attending to transfusions, morphine, oxygen, instrumental monitoring and checking wounds. The injured need reassurance more than anything else – more than they ever thought they would need. 'They're scared; they're pumped up; I have to be the voice of reason. I tell them, "I'm the flight medic. I'm going to take care of you all the way to the hospital."'

Balad has cared for thousands of patients in a single year and every month there are about 400 operations in three trailer operating rooms with forty ward beds and twenty intensive-care beds. Eight patients at a time can use lung-ventilating machines. The staffing structure tells the story of today's injuries – several general surgeons, four orthopaedic surgeons, a neurosurgeon, a chest surgeon, an eye surgeon, an oral surgeon, a facial surgeon and two hand surgeons, supported by nurses, technicians, medics, anaesthetists and radiologists. It is claimed that Balad Hospital can do anything that a major medical centre in the United States can do, except organ transplantation. According to a hospital commander:

> I have people fighting to get here so they can do this job. [Some of them] are
> the most highly skilled surgeons in the world and they are doing something

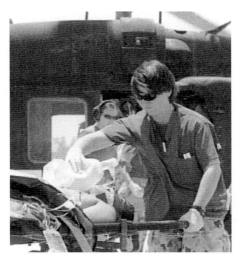

An anaesthetic nurse ventilates an urgent patient and assists in moving him to waiting transport, Iraq, 2004. (*Dr G. K. Bruce*)

that is so righteous. They know they'll never have the chance to do this again in their entire lives. So they don't want to leave.

Compared with Vietnam, a slightly higher rate of death in Iraq military hospitals is probably related to the fact that a greater number of the worst injured now actually reach hospital rather than die in the field. Combat surgeons report that most injuries are the result of IEDs, which produce more and worse injuries than ever seen before. Iraqis are also being injured by their own people and require care in an allied military hospital if they are to be treated at all.

Colonel W. D. Clouse and his colleagues have recently reported their experience with nearly 7,000 'battle-related' vascular (large blood vessel) injuries treated between 2004 and 2006 at Balad. As in all wars, most work is on limbs, while half of the remainder involves the neck and the rest involves the trunk. The remarkable statistic is that most patients are not Americans – they are Iraqi civilians, soldiers and police injured by Iraqi weapons in the hands of Iraqis. They include the very people who lay the bombs that kill and wound Allied troops. As in Afghanistan, surgeons treat Iraqis in the same trauma rooms as they treat their own men.

State-of-the-art first aid had been carried out on most of them at the point of injury before transfer to the specialist centre, much like the MASH rescue developed in the Second World War. Clouse reported that the majority had full repair of their blood vessels producing a halving of the amputation rate of similar injuries in Korea and Vietnam. The number of vascular injuries in Iraq and Afghanistan seems about twice that of Vietnam, but limb survival rates are much higher, probably because of the ultra-rapid evacuation to nearly ideal surgical conditions – often within minutes of injury.

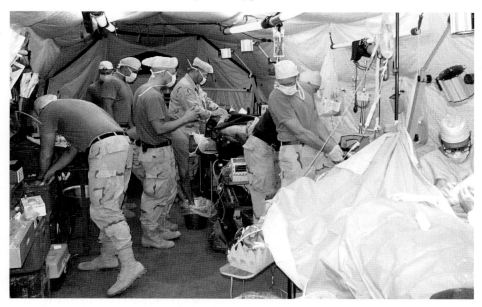

Three patients in an operating tent, Balad, 2005. Two (centre and rear) are being prepared and one (right foreground) is already undergoing an operation. (*Dr H. Stinger*)

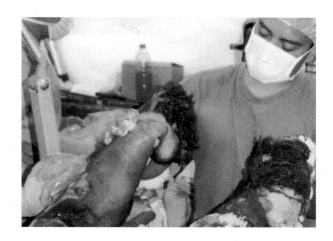

Destroyed lower legs from a typical ground-level IED explosion, Balad, Iraq. (*Dr G. Peoples*)

Nessen and his colleagues have recently published a remarkable surgical teaching atlas of current war injuries that shows the range of state-of-the-art equipment and procedures developed and employed in Iraq and Afghanistan today.

Zucchino reports that most surgeons say the same of their job as the great French surgeon, Baron Larrey, said of his during the Napoleonic Wars:

You're not the judge or jury in the emergency room – you are a doctor. It is irrelevant ... what a patient's status is. I am going to do what I'd do for an

American. You just don't see injuries like this in the US. I don't ever want
to see injuries like this ... I try not to think about a patient being a person
sometimes ... if you are thinking about him as somebody's son, it's very
difficult to take care of him ... sometimes it's not possible.

The ideal Forward Surgical Teams (FST) consist of three general surgeons, one
orthopaedic surgeon, two nurse anaesthetists, three general nurses, medics and
other support personnel. They provide mobile medical care much closer to the
military fronts than was ever the case in Vietnam. They have some laboratory
facilities, a portable ultrasound machine, monitors, ventilators and banks of
packed red blood cells.

Because X-rays are not available to the FSTs, surgeons diagnose most
fractures by touch or sight. The teams are equipped for six hours of post-
operative intensive care, with each team having four ventilated beds and
two operating tables. They travel in 'Humvees' (high-mobility multi-purpose
wheeled vehicles) that can also carry troops and armaments and act as
ambulances or scouts. They carry just enough equipment to salvage and
resuscitate the wounded in emergencies. The FSTs aim for damage control
rather than definitive repair. Surgery is limited to about two hours of acute
salvage procedures per case before the patient is shipped back by controlled
airspace or road to a Combat Support Hospital (CSH) for further care.

Some surgeons continue to question the idea of life-saving surgery and
resuscitation being done in front-line conditions where, apart from blood, only
limited equipment, communication and resources are available to them. They
see it as impractical to set up significant numbers of trauma centres in combat
zones when immediate, urgent evacuation might provide the greatest good
for the greatest number of injured men. Nonetheless, experience in Korea and
Vietnam clearly showed that MASH units are of crucial value in providing
expert forward expertise in all combat areas.

CSHs are also mobile units, but are much more substantial than the FSTs.
In 2004, there were two of them in Iraq providing 248 beds with six operating
tables. They are transported by air, tractor, trailer or ship and can be fully
functional within two days. After a few days in a CSH, the seriously wounded
are transferred to bases in Kuwait, Spain or Germany. US troops requiring
more than a month of treatment are transferred to the USA.

One airman in extremis from devastating injuries in a mortar attack in
Iraq was on an operating table at Walter Reed Army Hospital, Washington,
DC, thirty-six hours later. After weeks in intensive care and after multiple
operations, he survived. Injuries like his could not be managed quickly enough
in previous wars, but the cost can be high in every way. He lost one leg above
knee, the other near the hip, his right hand and part of his face. With such
states of survival, elemental questions are raised about how men and their
families can ever adapt to, let alone function with, such extreme, permanent

disability. Just as disturbingly, surgeons are reporting a large number of troops with blindness in one or both eyes. The combination of high survival rates and substantial, permanent incapacity presents enormous medical, logistical and economic challenges that will continue indefinitely.

Despite the stresses and risks of the job, many surgeons, private security men and 'contractors' choose to have multiple deployments in Iraq or Afghanistan. Clearly, there are some worthwhile incentives, apart from gaining experience, for them to leave home and go to live and work in danger and under constant stress. One young surgeon, who began his army service in 2001, had fulfilled the terms of a military scholarship to attend medical school and was deployed twice to Iraq. Four days before returning home from his second deployment, he was hit by a rocket-propelled grenade while making a telephone call to his family from a payphone in his barracks. He did not survive.

Karl Vick of the *Washington Post* Foreign Service described a macabre scene reflecting what he called, 'The Lasting Wounds of War':

Soldiers were lifted into the helicopters under a moonless sky, their bandaged heads grossly swollen by trauma, their forms silhouetted by ... medical monitors ... an orange screen registering blood pressure and heart rate ... a blue screen [measuring] pressure on the brain ... a grey [box] recording medicines pumping into the body and a respirator breathing the lungs.

More and more in Iraq, combat surgeons say, the wounds involve severe damage to the head and eyes, injuries that leave soldiers brain-damaged or blind, or both, and the doctors ... struggling against despair. The gravest wounds have been caused by roadside bombs, improvised explosives defying the protection of Kevlar helmets by blowing shrapnel and dirt upward into the face. In addition, fights with guerrillas have surged recently, causing a sharp rise in gunshot wounds to the vital areas not protected by body armor.

According to some reports, many soldiers in Iraq seem to complain less about being there than they do from a fear that the American public no longer support them as they once did. Even so, many veterans of the war return for two or three tours of duty. They often make the same observation – that Arabs tend not to fight 'stand-up' wars as the Americans do. They allow an invading army to capture the region and then attempt to pick them off until the occupiers go home. It has become a long and, perhaps, endless campaign of attrition and guerrilla warfare.

DEADLY TOOLS OF WAR

What follows are soldiers' words on things only they can know and feel. A marine is describing the weapons they use and how effectively they produce casualties. This is not just a technical account of weapons, but it tells of who is on both sides of the conflict. It describes how they think, who becomes involved voluntarily or involuntarily, how they suffer, how they respond, who treats them for what, and how the future looked to this experienced observer just a few years ago.

Recent criticisms of the value and morale of Allied forces is in sharp contrast with this soldier's account of the circumstances that he experienced in Iraq. Clearly, he learned a great deal about weapons used on both sides and the moods and methods of his opponents. He creates a pragmatic image of the totality of that war and how it feels to spend months in service in Ramada. These astounding, unclassified, verbatim observations in the field were first provided by Robin Hardy in 2005:

US Weapons

M-16 rifle: Thumbs down. Chronic jamming problems with the talcum powder like sand over there. The sand is everywhere. Jordan says you feel filthy 2 minutes after coming out of the shower. The M-4 carbine version is more popular because it's lighter and shorter, but it has jamming problems also. They like the ability to mount the various optical gun-sights and weapons lights on the piccaninny rails, but the weapon itself is not great in a desert environment. They all hate the 5.56-mm (.223) round. Poor penetration on the cinderblock structure common over there and even torso hits can't be reliably counted on to put the enemy down. Fun fact: Random autopsies on dead insurgents show a high level of opiate use.

M243 SAW (squad assault weapon): Light machine gun. Big thumbs down. Universally considered a piece of shit. Chronic jamming problems, most of which require partial disassembly (that's fun in the middle of a fire fight).

M9 Beretta 9-mm: Mixed bag. Good gun, performs well in desert environment; but they all hate the 9-mm cartridge. The use of handguns for self-defense is actually fairly common. Same old story on the 9-mm: bad guys hit multiple times and still in the fight.

Mossberg 12ga Military shotgun: Works well, used frequently for clearing houses to good effect.

M240 machine gun: Developed to replace the old M-60 (what a beautiful weapon that was!!). Thumbs up. Accurate, reliable, and the 7.62 round puts 'em down. Originally developed as a vehicle mounted weapon, more and more are being dismounted and taken into the field by infantry. The 7.62 round chews up the structure over there.

M2.50 cal heavy machine gun: Thumbs way, way up. 'Ma deuce' is still worth her considerable weight in gold. The ultimate fight stopper, puts their dicks in the dirt every time. The most coveted weapon in-theater.

.45 cal pistol: Thumbs up. Still the best pistol round out there. Everybody authorized to carry a sidearm is trying to get their hands on one. With few exceptions, can reliably be expected to put 'em down with a torso hit. The special ops guys (who are doing most of the pistol work) use the HK military model and supposedly love it. The old government model .45's are being re-issued en masse.

M-14: Thumbs up. They are being re-issued in bulk, mostly in a modified version to special ops guys. Modifications include lightweight Kevlar stocks and low power red dot or ACOG sights. Very reliable in the sandy environment, and they love the 7.62 round.

Barrett .50 cal sniper rifle: Thumbs way up. Spectacular range and accuracy and hits like a freight train. Used frequently to take out vehicle suicide bombers (we actually stop a lot of them) and barricaded enemy. Definitely here to stay.

M24 sniper rifle: Thumbs up. Mostly in .308 but some in .300 mag. Heavily modified Remington 700s. Great performance. Snipers have been used heavily to great effect. Rumor has it that a marine sniper on his third tour in Anbar province has actually exceeded Carlos Hathcock's record for confirmed kills with OVER 100.

New body armor: Thumbs up. Relatively light at approx. 6 lbs and can reliably be expected to soak up small shrapnel and even will stop an AK-47 round. The bad news: hot as shit to wear, almost unbearable in the summer heat (which averages over 120 degrees). Also, the enemy now goes for head shots whenever possible. All the stuff about the 'old' (but not the 'new') body armor making our guys vulnerable to the I.E.D.s is a non-starter. The I.E.D. explosions are enormous and body armor doesn't make any difference at all in most cases.

Night Vision and Infrared Equipment: Thumbs way up. Spectacular performance. Our guys see in the dark and own the night, period. Very little enemy action after evening prayers. More and more enemy being whacked at night during movement by hunter-killer teams.

Lights: Thumbs up. Most of the weapon mounted and personal lights are Surefire's, and the troops love 'em. Invaluable for night urban operations.

'Bad Guy' Weapons

AK47 rifle: The entire country is an arsenal. Works better in the desert than the M16 and the .308 Russian round kills reliably. PKM belt fed light machine guns are also common and effective. Luckily, the enemy mostly shoots poorly. Undisciplined 'spray and pray' type fire. However, they are seeing more and more precision weapons, especially sniper rifles (Iran, again). Fun fact: Captured enemy have apparently marveled at the marksmanship of our guys and how hard they fight. They are apparently told in Jihad school that the Americans rely solely on technology, and can be easily beaten in close quarters combat for their lack of toughness. Let's just say they know better now.

RPG (rocket-propelled grenade): Probably the infantry weapon most feared by our guys. Simple, reliable and as common as dog shit. The enemy responded to our uparmored Humvees by aiming at the windshields, often at point blank range. Still killing a lot of our guys.

Improvised Explosive Devices: The biggest killer of all. Can be anything from old Soviet anti-armor mines to jury rigged artillery shells. A lot found in Jordan's area were in abandoned cars. The enemy would take 2 or 3 155-mm artillery shells and wire them together. Most were detonated by cell phone, and the explosions are enormous. You're not safe in any vehicle, even an M1 tank. Driving is by far the most dangerous thing our guys do over there. Lately, they are much more sophisticated 'shape charges' (Iranian) specifically designed to penetrate armor. Fact: Most of the ready made IEDs are supplied by Iran, who is also providing terrorists (Hezbollah types) to train the insurgents in their use and tactics. That's why the attacks have been so deadly lately. Their concealment methods are ingenious, the latest being shape charges in Styrofoam containers spray painted to look like the cinderblocks that litter all Iraqi roads. We find about 40 per cent before they detonate, and the bomb disposal guys are unsung heroes of this war, they and the surgeons.

Mortars and rockets: Very prevalent. The Soviet-era 122-mm rockets (with an 18 kilometre range) are becoming more prevalent. One of the marine's NCOs lost a leg to one. These weapons cause a lot of damage 'inside the wire'. Marine's base was hit almost daily his entire time there by mortar and rocket fire, often at night to disrupt sleep patterns and cause fatigue (it did). More of a psychological weapon than anything else. The enemy mortar teams would jump out of vehicles, fire a few rounds, and then haul ass in a matter of seconds.

Bad guy technology: Simple yet effective. Most communication is by cell and satellite phones, and also by email on laptops. They use handheld GPS units for navigation and 'Google earth' for overhead views of our positions. Their weapons are good, if not fancy, and prevalent. Their explosives and bomb technology is TOP OF THE LINE. Night vision is rare. They are very careless with their equipment and the captured GPS units and laptops are treasure troves of Intel when captured.

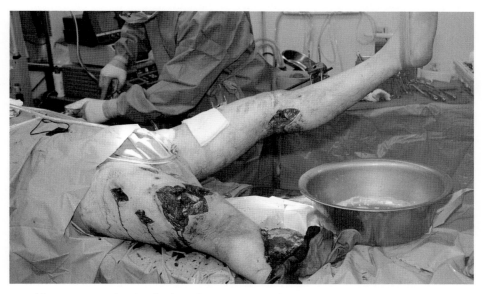

IED blast injuries of right thigh and amputation of right leg below knee; there is also a large left knee injury affecting nerves and blood vessels. (*Dr G. K. Bruce*)

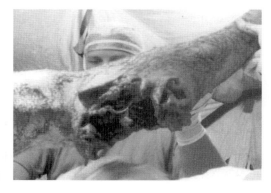

Shredded elbow demanding amputation, Iraq. (*Dr G. Peoples*)

Who Are The Bad Guys?

Most of the carnage is caused by the (Zarqawi) Al Qaeda group. They keep the surgeons too busy. They operate mostly in Anbar province (Fallujah and Ramadi). These are mostly 'foreigners', non-Iraqi Sunni Arab Jihadists from all over the Muslim world (and Europe). Most enter Iraq through Syria (with, of course, the knowledge and complicity of the Syrian govt.) and then travel down the 'rat line' which is the trail of towns along the Euphrates River that we've been hitting hard for the last few months.

Some are virtually untrained young Jihadists that often end up as suicide bombers or in 'sacrifice squads'. Most, however, are hard core terrorists from all the usual suspects (Al Qaeda, Hezbollah, Hamas, etc.). These are the guys running around murdering civilians en masse and cutting heads off. The Chechens (many of whom are Caucasian) are supposedly the most ruthless and the best fighters. (They have been fighting the Russians for years.) In the Baghdad area and south, most of the insurgents are Iranian inspired (and led) Iraqi Shiites. The Iranian Shiia have been very adept at infiltrating the Iraqi local govt., the police forces and the Army. They have had a massive spy and agitator network there since the Iran-Iraq war in the early 1980s. Most of the Saddam loyalists were killed, captured or gave up long ago.

Bad Guy Tactics

When they are engaged [in battle] on an infantry level they get their asses kicked every time. Brave, but stupid. Suicidal Banzai-type charges were very common earlier in the war and still occur. They will literally sacrifice 8–10 man teams in suicide squads by sending them screaming and firing AKs and RPGs directly at our bases just to probe the defenses. They get mowed down like grass every time. (see the M2 and M240 above).

Jordan's base was hit like this often. When engaged, they have a tendency to flee to the same building, probably for what they think will be a glorious last stand. Instead, we call in air and that's the end of that more often than not. These hole-ups are referred to as Alpha Whiskey Romeo's (Allah's Waiting Room). We have the laser guided ground-air thing down to a science. The fast mover's, mostly Marine F-18s, are taking an ever increasing toll on the enemy. When caught out in the open, the helicopter gunships and AC-130 Spectre gunships cut them to ribbons with cannon and rocket fire, especially at night. Interestingly, artillery is hardly used at all.

Other Fun Facts

The enemy death toll is supposedly between 45 and 50,000. That is why we're seeing less and less infantry attacks and more IED, suicide bomber stuff.

The new strategy is simple: attrition. The insurgent tactic most frustrating is their use of civilian non-combatants as cover. They know we do all we can to avoid civilian casualties and therefore schools, hospitals and (especially) Mosques are locations where they meet, stage for attacks, cache weapons and ammo and flee to when engaged. They have absolutely no regard whatsoever for civilian casualties. They will terrorize locals and murder without hesitation anyone believed to be sympathetic to the Americans or the new Iraqi government. Kidnapping of family members (especially children) is common to influence people they are trying to influence but can't reach, such as local govt. officials, clerics, tribal leaders, etc.).

The Iraqi's are a mixed bag. Some fight well, others aren't worth a shit. Most do okay with American support. Finding leaders is hard, but they are getting better. It is widely viewed that Zarqawi's use of suicide bombers, en masse, against the civilian population was a serious tactical mistake. Many Iraqi's were galvanized and the caliber of recruits in the Army and the police forces went up, along with their motivation. It also led to an exponential increase in good intelligence because the Iraqi's are sick of the insurgent attacks against civilians. The Kurds are solidly pro-American and fearless fighters.

Morale among our guys is very high. The medical people see to that. The troops not only believe they are winning, but that they are winning decisively. They are stunned and dismayed by what they see in the America press, whom they almost universally view as against them. The embedded reporters are despised and distrusted. They are inflicting casualties at a rate of 20–1 and then see things like 'Are we losing in Iraq?' on TV and the print media. For the most part, we are satisfied with equipment, food and leadership. Bottom line though, and they all say this, there are not enough guys there to drive the final stake through the heart of the insurgency, primarily because there aren't enough troops in-theater to shut down the borders with Iran and Syria. The Iranians and the Syrians just can't stand the thought of Iraq being an American ally (with, of course, permanent US bases there).

DEVELOPING SAFER HUMVEES

We love death. The US loves life. That is the big difference between us.

– Osama bin Laden, 2001

Despite their great versatility, Humvees (high-mobility-multi-purpose-wheeled-vehicles) have sustained a large number of devastating attacks in Iraq and Afghanistan. They have been modified many times, largely at the instigation of surgeons who treat wounded crews. Their original value was for lightweight, cross-country mobility and they were not armoured as fighting vehicles. Following attacks on them, they were soon adapted for active combat but have become enticing targets. They frequently carry medical personnel and some are fitted for urgent life-saving surgery.

Recently, up-armoured vehicles, as suggested by surgical commanders, have incorporated an optional protection kit which adds a ton to the weight of the standard vehicle but reduces its vulnerability. Steel plating and armoured windows around the cabin offer better protection against small-arms fire and shrapnel and additional plating beneath the engine and cabin floor resists many high explosives. Up-armoured or not, all vehicles remain targets for cluster bombs and grenades thrown through their windows and for mines and rockets at ground level. In military parlance, these weapons leave a much larger 'footprint' of destruction than other explosives.

Despite improved armour, improvised bombs remain the major killers of Humvee crews. The challenge is to outwit the bomber before he outwits the targets. Many crews spread filled sandbags on the cabin floor to help protect them from 'blast' from below – exactly the same injury as was first described after explosions between the decks of ships. 'Blast lung' is especially treacherous because of its delayed onset of symptoms and need for prolonged lung ventilation, but the concussive effect is usually associated with fumes and burns. As well as damage by the blast wave to the brain, bowel and ears, low-level shrapnel extends the injuries to the lower body and compounds surgical difficulties.

The basic Humvee has lost much of its value with the increasing ingenuity of those who manufacture IEDs. Its low ground clearance, flat bottom and fragile panels and floor have been exploited by insurgents who use devices containing quantities of explosive ranging from soda-can size up to that of a motor van. They can contain shells, mortars, fertiliser, fuel, metal scrap and armour-piercing arrows on or near the roadside, used singly or in chains.

Following surgical, military and political pressures, MRAP (mine-resistant, ambush-protected) vehicles are now being demanded for any dangerous patrol and combat mission. These come into service at up to $1 million each – three-to-five times the cost of a standard Humvee. They rely on very heavy armour, a higher carriage and a heavy-duty, V-shaped floor to deflect blast away from the vehicle and impart greater resistance to the effects of IEDs. They have been described as 'tanks on wheels' able to carry up to twelve troops, but with slower ground speeds than earlier models.

In further defensive measures, the US Army is intensifying production of electronic jamming devices which work against remote trigger-systems such as phones, remote door-openers and radios – often used at long range. The battle for higher soldier survival rates goes on at vastly increased expense, but surgeons, the military and the public will no longer accept the fragility of the early Humvees for all duties. Thomas J. Nelson and his surgical colleagues recently analysed the morbid effects of blast from terrorist bombs in Iraq where they saw the same types of injuries as occurred in Oklahoma City, Madrid, Istanbul, Israel, London, Bali and, more recently, Morocco, India, Pakistan and elsewhere.

The major immediate first-aid problems are shock, penetrating head injuries and multiple limb fractures. Victims with two or more of those effects have a 90 per cent mortality rate. At the time of injury, most troops in Iraq, as in Afghanistan, were wearing Kevlar helmets and body-armour with protective inserts for armpits, groins and neck. Ballistic eyewear was not mandatory. The least injured were transported by helicopter to more convenient areas of care. Wherever possible, resuscitation of the most badly injured was attempted immediately. Of eighteen consecutive blast victims seen in late 2004, four had been killed immediately and five others died soon after, regardless of all immediate measures. That left only nine who survived long enough to be evacuated to a higher level of care. The study concluded that all patients with early onset of shock would die, whatever was done for them, most within an hour of wounding.

Clearly, blast injuries will increase wherever urban terrorists operate because they favour the bombing of enclosed public transport vehicles rather than open spaces. Wounds are mostly associated with penetrations of the head and trunk and significant burns, rather than any other form of injury. Inevitably, the closer the victim is to the source of blast, the worse the injuries.

Even more macabre features of suicide bombing have recently been noted in Iraq when body parts of the bombers have been blasted into the tissues of victims to impart a bizarre form of disease inoculation. As a result, some casualties have later developed hepatitis or HIV antibodies. Additionally, pregnant women, even though distant from explosions, have sustained foetal injury, uterine rupture or premature delivery.

Dr Amy Vertrees and other surgeons from the Walter Reed Army Medical Centre in Washington have recently reported their experience of twenty-nine young soldiers who had been crushed by bomb-blasted Humvees, or by violent compression from collisions, air crashes or building collapse. All were given emergency treatment in Iraq, 'packaged' for evacuation within a few days, bussed to the Ramstein Air Base for the same grade of intensive care in C-17 transports at 35,000 feet for eight hours and delivered to Dr Vertrees' group. Admittedly, the injuries were more severe than would be expected in civilian life but the lessons are universally applicable.

They confirmed an aspect of blast injury that was described originally by Russian surgeons in Afghanistan in 2001. So severe and sudden was the initial state of shock from multiple wounds that men required rapid blood transfusions of up to twice their normal 10 to 12 pint blood content. Without that extreme measure, their shock rapidly became uncontrollable with kidney failure and death. In each case, these men owed their survival to the immediate medical care given by 'buddies' and medics, frequently deep within combat zones.

Humvee casualties of Iraq and Afghanistan are typified by Tim Post's report on Minnesota Public Radio about a soldier who survived a massive blast in a Humvee in Iraq and was finally sent home with brain damage and one leg shorter than the other. He had been on patrol when an IED killed the driver instantly and left the soldier trapped in the back of the vehicle. Another soldier was blasted out into the desert, dead:

> I remember most of being in Iraq, but I don't remember the day of the attack or a couple of days before … I don't want to remember anything that happened to me that day. If I remember, it'll keep me awake at night. Then I'm not going to be able to sleep and I'll cry my eyes out. We drove over an IED. It was a shell – pretty damn big. We drove over the top of it and it blew up. It blew the Humvee up into the air and it went off into the desert. They heard me moaning and opened up the back door. My name [on his uniform] was covered up [and] my face was full of blood.

He was bleeding heavily from serious shrapnel injuries to his head and legs. After stabilisation, he was sent to a military hospital in Germany for a couple of months before his transfer to the Walter Reed Hospital in Washington for convalescence. When he returned to the family farm eight months later, he could walk around the house unaided, but his brain injury was more trouble than his leg. Speech therapy has helped but conversation is difficult. He says his injuries would have killed him in other wars and wonders if he might have been a better off. Others ask the same question.

Michael Georgy has given an expert account of practical measures for avoiding suspicious vehicles in the precincts of hospitals, health clinics, ambulances, first-aid posts and police stations. He estimates that Iraqi and imported suicide bombers have killed thousands of civilians and injured many more. No medical team is immune to the same risks. Limiting the dangers of terrorists depends on rapidly identifying suspicious vehicles and individuals and adopting a very pro-active response to them.

Georgy's recommended principles of defence are universally applicable:

While US marines in Iraq might have their tanks, they say they are helpless in the face of the increasing sophistication of suicide bombers and their rickety cars. They [suicide bombers] used to drive cars alone but now they appear in groups of three to fool everyone. This is one of our biggest concerns. It is hard to tell these cars apart from other ones. They are getting more sophisticated. They pack explosives in old cars that are ... difficult to detect.

Marines ... in some of the most powerful tanks ever made ... may have trouble spotting suicide bombers because they look like any other motorist; by the time they are detected, it's too late. You have about ten seconds to react. [Our] tanks are designed for open terrain. In Fallujah a car can just cross a street and hit you.

[We] ... wave them away. Then shoot their tires. Then shoot their headlights. Then shoot them. Blinking headlights or vehicles making U-turns raise suspicion and then weapons appear at the windows of our vehicles. How can you prepare for a car just coming at you?

Marines may have increased their vigilance but they are fearful wherever they are, struggling to understand why their enemies would want to blow themselves up and why surgeons have to treat them when they fail. One of them told Georgy:

I try not to think about it. I have seen what they can do to a seven-tonne truck and ... the guys are scared. I try to talk to them and help them or they go to the chaplain. In a way, I can see these people are defending their country. I hope I never have to defend my country that way. In fact, I know I won't.

OPERATION IRAQI FREEDOM

In the 1920s, the Italians were the first to land troops and medical staff by parachute, soon followed by the use of gliders and helicopters by Germany, Britain, India and the United States. The first large deployment of airborne military specialists was in Korea. It was repeated in Vietnam for large-scale transportation of men and equipment and for evacuation of the injured. Because of their high mobility and speed, parachutists and their equipment remain essential parts of all modern armies and their surgical forces.

A distinguished American surgeon, Lieutenant-Colonel Harry K. Stinger, has given me permission to reproduce some of his report published in *The Bulletin of the American College of Surgeons* in March 2004. It serves to reflect the exceptional courage and expertise of Stinger's group. The opinions expressed in the article are those of Colonel Stinger and do not necessarily reflect the views of *The Bulletin*, the US Army Medical Department, the US Army or the US Department of Defence. The following is an edited version of his remarkable paper, which describes the deployment of nine paratrooper-surgeons and medics, with their equipment, into Bashur airfield in northern Iraq on 26 March 2003. Two Humvee cargo trucks, loaded with enough equipment to perform ten resuscitative procedures, were dropped with the surgeons who were accompanied by paratroopers armed with machine-guns, mortars and grenades.

As commander of the 250th Forward Surgical Team (FST), Colonel Stinger was accompanied by three other surgeons who had intensively prepared themselves in Italy before proceeding to Iraq. The jump was described as a 'routine' mission. The team carried twenty units of type O-negative packed red blood-cells strapped in the front passenger seats of two parachute-rigged Humvees.

The parachuting of vehicles and artillery from powered aircraft has largely replaced the glider forces of the Second World War, which usually needed to land to discharge their cargo of men and their equipment, jeeps and artillery. Colonel Stinger's was the first forward surgical team to parachute directly into a combat zone since the Second World War. Here is some of what he wrote:

> The need for a small, easy-to-insert surgical capability became evident during the US-led invasion of Grenada in 1983. At that time, the smallest army unit that could perform surgery was a Mobile Army Surgical Hospital (MASH). Because of its … weight and size, the first MASH did not make it into Grenada until four days after the invasion started. This prompted the army to develop the FST to meet the need for a small, readily deployed surgical team that could perform resuscitative … surgical procedures on soldiers from the moment the fighting began. By 1986, Army surgical squads were organised and actually jumped in with paratroops during the invasion of Panama in 1989. These small squads had to wait for aircraft to land before they could access their operating tables, anaesthesia machines and other heavy equipment.

Airborne surgical teams (FST) were first used by the US Army in the early 1990s and introduced the principle of parachuting equipment into combat

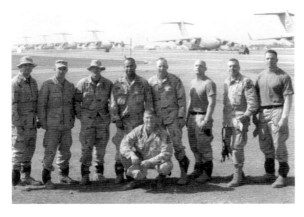

Colonel Harry Stinger (second from right) and the members of his team of paratrooper surgeons and medics, parachuted into Iraq with their equipment in 2003.
(*Dr H. Stinger*)

areas ahead of surgical teams in order to provide immediate access to life-saving materials within the 'golden hour' of greatest survival chance. Hardware was parachuted or delivered by tactical aircraft that landed in the vicinity of the combat zone:

> Each FST in Operation Iraqi Freedom consisted of 20 personnel: four surgeons, five nurses, a medical operations officer and 10 enlisted medics who specialise not only in trauma surgical procedures but also in the pre- and post-operative care of combat casualties. All surgeons and nurses were board-certified in their respective specialties and used state-of-the-art equipment and techniques to provide the best trauma care to troops who happened to be injured in the line of duty.

According to Dr Robert Rush:

> By far, the most useful item was the Sonosite portable ultrasound ... [This] was very useful as [an objective] triage tool, as the injured paratroopers we work on have tremendous physiologic reserve. This diminishes the reliance on routine vital signs in making triage decisions. We also used the Sonosite to screen for traumatic pseudo-aneurysms, assess the adequacy of vascular repairs and eventually even assess congenital heart defects in young Iraqi children.

Among the equipment carried by the FST were tent shelters, anaesthetic machines, laboratory equipment and oxygen concentrators replacing pressurised gas tanks:

> All of the team's equipment was fully transportable on just six cargo Humvees. In contrast, it would take a minimum of four standard 18-wheelers to transport a MASH but the FST was not a complete hospital. It is just the surgical section of a hospital that performed resuscitative, as opposed to definitive, surgical procedures designed to render the casualty transportable to the rear-area hospital. Because of its small size and proximity to the front-line, every member of the team had to be an initiative-taking, 150 per cent performer all of the time. Potential team members were carefully selected to screen out those who thought they could get by with doing the minimum. Excellence in trauma surgery and combat casualty care is what we were all about.

Once airfields were secured, it took Stinger's team less than two hours to set up the tents which served as pre-operative preparation areas, operating rooms and post-operative, intensive-care facilities. By that time, cargo planes had landed and delivered the rest of the team's personnel and additional equipment.

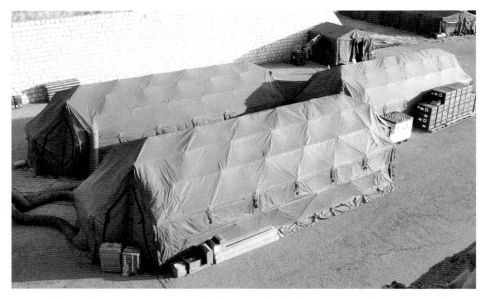

A portable canvas operating tent, Balad, Iraq; note the large air-conditioning conduits to the left. (*Dr H. Stinger*)

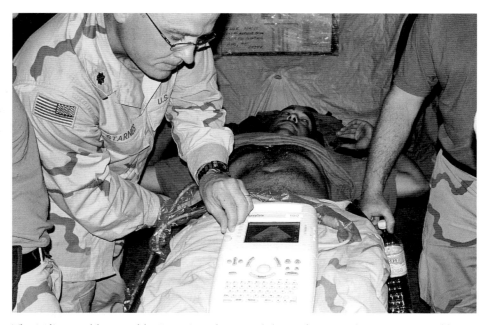

The indispensable portable 'Sonosite' ultrasound device for immediate screening of bones and soft tissues. (*Dr H. Stinger*)

The 250th FST initially set up near an abandoned but usable airstrip in north-east Iraq named Bashur airfield. That remote airfield was situated in Kurdish-held territory between two mountain ranges. Fortunately, the Kurdish militia had succeeded in subduing all hostile forces in and round the area, so that there was no enemy fire on the drop zone when the 173rd Airborne troops jumped.

Build-up of combat power in and round the airfield proceeded and in mid-April the mission changed and the 173rd Airborne Brigade had to repack their equipment and convoy 178 kilometres south to the Iraqi oil-rich city of Kirkuk. The city was of vital strategic importance and it was critical that American forces quickly take control to avert civil unrest. Stinger's team had to be divided into two echelons again in order to preserve surgical capability during the convoy. A five-member team remained behind to care for a soldier with a gunshot wound to the hip awaiting evacuation to Germany.

When the team reunited later on a military airfield in Kirkuk, it was fully operational again and able to take care of American soldiers, Coalition forces, Iraqi civilians and enemy combatants. The surgical procedures carried out were comprehensive, including management of fractures, repair of major blood vessel and chest injuries, injuries from shrapnel and gunshot, knife wounds, burns and blunt trauma:

> Not every surgeon has had the opportunity to operate to the sound of explosions and small arms fire in the background. Kirkuk turned out to be a coalition success story. The 173rd Airborne paratroopers set up safe houses within Kirkuk and immediately began backing up the local police and establishing order and civil functions. Terrorist attacks were minimised. I believe the people of Kirkuk were very happy to have Americans there and are very thankful that we freed them from a miserable dictator.
>
> After the combat operations of the war were over, the FSTs took on the civil affairs job of helping to reinforce the medical infrastructure within the city. This required hospital assessments of critical shortages. While touring these facilities, members of the team received occasional indirect enemy fire but remained undeterred.
>
> Enthusiastic to meet their surgical colleagues in war-torn Iraq, the FST surgeons then made liaison trips to the two largest hospitals in Kirkuk, Saddam Hospital and Kirkuk General Hospital. The Kirkuk physicians resented having Saddam's name affiliated with one of the institutions and immediately renamed it Azadi Hospital (Azadi translates as 'freedom' in the Kurdish language). Kirkuk's ethnic composition is 60 per cent Kurdish, 20 per cent Turkish and 20 per cent Arab.

Colonel Stinger has great admiration for the medical sergeants who worked with his team. He regarded them as the backbone of the army, men able to train soldiers and maintain the team's programme. He also admired the brave Iraqi surgeons who stayed in Kirkuk during the war.

As foreign combatants begin to leave Iraq to its own 'democratic' devices and may soon begin a similar, staged withdrawal from Afghanistan, these countries will find the pressures of maintaining their own surgical services difficult. Medical installations which are free and freely available and capable of almost any service possible in major hospitals in America and Europe will be sorely missed.

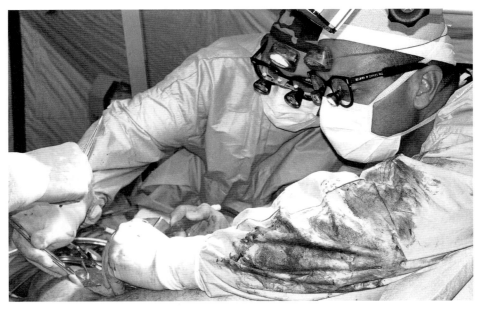

A difficult view of a deep wound despite using headlights and magnifying lenses. (*Dr H. Stinger*)

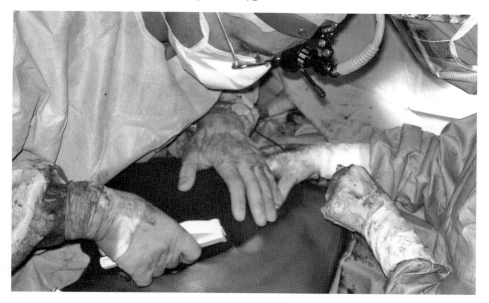

The rapid closure of abdominal skin by staples at the end of an operation. (*Dr H. Stinger*)

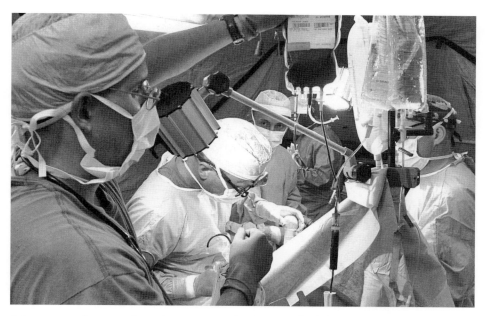

A busy operating team in action: an anaesthetist is on the left, surgeons are in the centre, and blood transfusion is running. (*Dr H. Stinger*)

CHAPTER 16

Women and War Injuries

A female air force officer observed that the Iraq war seemed to have answered questions about America's response to seeing women return home in bandages and body bags. 'There have been casualties, men and women, and we grieve for them. But I think we have gotten beyond the point where losing a daughter is somehow worse than losing a son.'

– Dave Moniz, 'Female amputees make clear that all troops are on front line,'
USA Today, 28 April 2005

Eight American nurses died in combat zones in Vietnam. Although hundreds died in previous wars, most of them were working in rear areas and died of diseases and injuries unrelated to combat. By 2008, 35 American servicewomen had died in combat in Iraq, 271 had been wounded and 6 had lost limbs – some multiple. It is the first time that large numbers of females have been involved or died in combat areas. A female amputee from Vietnam said: 'If you lost a limb in Vietnam, you were automatically discharged. The big thing [today] is to show what your capabilities are.' Another Vietnam leg amputee, now a retired male judge, says those who lose limbs have to go through adjustments that most people can't imagine. One of the most difficult is getting used to people staring. He suspects that it will be even more difficult for women who are scarred.

An American nurse who cared for insurgents as well as Coalition forces in Baghdad left a husband and children back home while she made her contribution. She and eleven other unarmed military nurses worked around the clock in a seventy-five-bed ward of a field hospital.

Some Iraqi patients threw urine and faeces and spat on them, one female was actually bitten and three nurses were sexually assaulted. By general American standards, the nurses felt that they had not been able to give good patient care, but believed they saved a lot of lives in their four months service there. One wrote, 'Some we could, and some we couldn't [save]. And then we cried. [It was] the most meaningful thing I ever did, and the most horrible. I carry mental scars that I hope will heal.'

The nurses each worked seventy-two hours a week, frequently under attack by missiles. Each of them was responsible for about fifteen patients, including

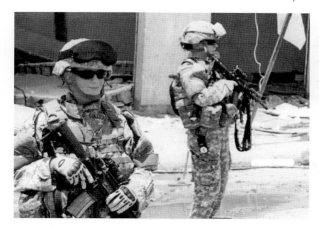

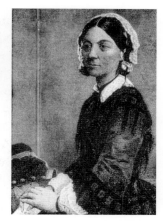

Above left: Armed and protected: an American female combat team in Iraq, 2007. (*US Army*)

Above right: The Crimean War's Florence Nightingale, perhaps the world's first 'medic'. (*Wikipedia*)

children and infants, many of whom had amputations from explosions, complicated chest injuries and other major wounds. A few had survived drowning.

One female lieutenant in the military police was working in Iraq when a rocket-propelled grenade exploded inside her Humvee. Her right arm was almost ripped off her body and the front passenger's right arm was severed completely. She shouted to her driver to, 'Get out of the kill zone!'

For six days surgeons fought the decision to amputate her arm, but they were defeated by spreading tissue-death and dangerous infection. After becoming an amputee, she had to think about what jobs she could do after leaving the army.

Her story might once have caused a debate over women being exposed to ground fighting but the facts of war have overtaken that question. She is often asked if women should be so heavily involved in fighting. 'Women in combat are not really an issue,' she says. 'It is happening. Everyone pretty much acknowledges there are no [true] rear battle areas any more [just as there is] no forward line of troops.' Iraq is not that sort of war and future wars will probably never be same as in the past.

In many cases, women are barred from the most hazardous positions such as in infantry, special operations, commandos, tank crews and where they would be exposed to typical front-line dangers, but they are allowed to fly fighter jets, serve as military police and fill other jobs that place them at high risk. With front-line and rearward troops sharing the same dangers in guerrilla wars in Iraq and Afghanistan, the military's wish to regulate risk is difficult or impossible to satisfy.

The most severely injured of the surviving female amputees from Iraq is Crystal Davis, a National Guard pilot who lost both legs when a rocket-propelled grenade hit her helicopter near Balad. Her right leg is amputated above the knee and her left leg below the knee. She believes she survived simply because the heat of the explosion coagulated her leg wounds and prevented her from bleeding to death while her co-pilot landed the aircraft. Without such luck or emergency aid, those injuries would have killed her from blood loss in a matter of minutes.

Five months later, she was learning again how to perform daily activities and to walk with fitted prostheses. For most who lose limbs, the recovery time before obtaining independent living again is about a year. Her husband supports her ambition to resume flying helicopters. A large number of severely wounded service members of both sexes have returned to active duty after amputations because their experiences can help others. Women remember a man who resumed flying jets after he lost a leg in a motorcycle accident. But he had discovered that an amputee has more difficulty in getting approval for combat flying these days than Douglas Bader, RAF air ace, did in the Second World War. The rules just do not allow it.

During her eight months of recovery at Walter Reed, a staff sergeant who lost part of her left arm when an improvised bomb exploded near her Humvee befriended other women who helped her cope. Her greatest difficulty was to learn to dress and eat with one real hand and one artificial one. The injury motivated her to attend school to become an army nurse. She has often noticed a particular difference among amputees. Men care much less about their appearance and many of them got around the hospital without wearing their artificial limbs. Women won't do that, she said, 'I just don't think America is ready to see a woman without an arm.'

Many women who worked in operating rooms, first aid, rescue helicopters and general hospital nursing have reported persistent nightmares after returning home from active service. There are no surprises there, as many of

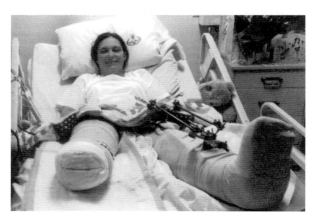

The heroic Crystal Davis. An IED explosion in Iraq caused her right lower limb to be amputated and a compound fracture in her left thigh; the left thigh has an external fixation device to immobilise the fracture during convalescence at Landstuhl, Germany. (*US Defense Department*)

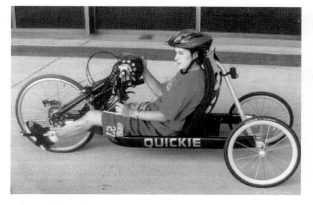
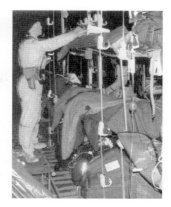

Above left: The amazing Crystal Davis undergoing intensive rehabilitation in the United States. (*US Defense Department*)

Above right: Patients on a flight to US Army Hospital, Landstuhl, with an armed nurse in attendance. (*Dr G. Peoples*)

them saw women and children killed by bombs, civilians shot, people almost disintegrated from bombs and even worse things – hard for civilians to imagine. They hoped they had been good soldiers, but it was difficult for them to resume normal domestic life with their families and children. Almost one in five of them has had a stress disorder treated in later life but a few yearn to do it all again in Iraq or Afghanistan. None of them witnessed any maltreatment of prisoners as was highly publicised from Abu Ghraib Prison, but some of them remember insults thrown at wounded suicide bombers by badly injured Americans.

At 2 p.m. on most days, a medical flight from the Balad Hospital airfield in Iraq to Landstuhl Military Hospital in Germany carries nurses, physicians, surgeons, respiratory therapists and others who care for severely injured men and women ready for evacuation from Iraq after a few days. On arrival, ambulances will be queued up to carry the wounded to the US Army hospital for further treatment. Men know that if they can make it that far, they are probably going to live, regardless of their injuries. Landstuhl takes up to 2,000 admissions a year and more than a quarter of them continue to need intensive care when they arrive. No soldier's life has been lost in transit to Germany. Some flights carry captured Iraqis who have been treated by army staff and need specialised treatment before returning to Iraq. One of them covered his heart with his right hand as an indication of respect and said through a translator, 'Your hospitals and staff are known throughout Iraq as angels of mercy.'

CHAPTER 17

The Human Costs of War

We saw the lightning, and that was the guns and then we heard the rain falling and that was the blood and when we came to get in the crops, it was dead men that we reaped.

– Harriet Tubman, *Divided Houses*, L. C. Sizer, 1992

The vast majority of those physically injured in war are treated by surgeons. Omissions and inaccuracies in the official records of armies make the counting of military dead and wounded imprecise, but a reasonable estimate is that more than 10 million soldiers were killed on the battlefields of the First World War and 30 million others were wounded or 'became missing' forever. One half of all enlisted troops had been injured or killed by the end of the war and in one year alone, there were nearly 100,000 British casualties just in Europe.

In 1914, the British Expeditionary Force consisted of only 150,000 professionals. Within a year, there were 200,000 and, by the end of 1914, over 1 million men and boys had joined up. Although many were poorly trained and short of equipment, Britain aimed to have an army of 2 million by the end of that war but actually achieved nearly 5 million, a quarter of the total male population.

The contributions of medical and surgical care in relieving the huge burdens of human damage in the world wars were enormous. Britain and its Empire suffered about a million deaths in the First World War and there were 2 million 'officially' wounded (from all causes) who were treated by doctors and nurses somewhere. The great majority of them survived. France and Russia suffered almost twice those numbers of casualties. A combination of Italian, American, Austro-Hungarian and Turkish forces in the First World War had over 7 million dead and 20 million wounded.

If the American Civil War was really 'the end of the middle ages' of battle surgery's evolution, the First World War was a threshold beyond which 'modern' medicine and surgery improved at a rate never before thought possible. In later wars, the salvage of life has increased unbelievably, meaning that the numbers of the permanently disabled have greatly increased. In other words, it is more difficult to kill a man now than ever before, but that means more and more disabled troops survive.

The French were the first to use chemical weapons in the form of tear gas, although the Germans soon followed. By 1915, the Germans had released 168 tons of chlorine gas to be carried by favourable winds across the Allied lines. Unfortunately for those in the path of the gas clouds, adequate masks and other protective equipment were not available for at least a year. As if chlorine was not bad enough, mustard and phosphorus gases were introduced by Germany in 1917 and about 200,000 of the Commonwealth forces were injured or killed by gas alone. Between all the warring nations, 1.3 million men were permanently gas affected.

As a smaller contributor to these tragic statistics of the First World War, Australia had about half a million enlistments, most of whom served overseas. About 54,000 were killed and 17,000 were gassed. Overall, more than one half of all those who enlisted became casualties of some sort, or were missing forever.

Before including a man's name on a casualty list, it is crucial for armies to try to identify him beyond reasonable doubt by full name, regimental number, unit and a statement of what happened to him. For ethical and record-keeping purposes, surgical systems, in particular, want to know whom they are treating, especially the mortally wounded, even if they are the enemy. Other men cannot or will not communicate, either because of, or despite of, their injuries. Some choose to remain anonymous and of doubtful affiliation and a significant number of others call themselves mercenaries or contractors. Any information is better than none and the next of kin of the wounded are urgently sought, even if never found. All armies try to limit the number of graves of 'unknown soldiers'. There are already enough imponderables without adding such permanent fixtures.

Whenever and wherever wars are fought, the most accurate estimates of mortality still come from medical and hospital reports, especially when surgery has been followed by a soldier's temporary immobilisation or death. Among the many factors leading to ambiguity in counting battle deaths are multiple reporting of single incidents, deaths of unknown cause, information withheld on 'security' grounds, disorientated men sent home to die, men hiding from their old lives and those dying of a 'disease' or unknown cause but unrelated to combat. It is little wonder, therefore, that there have always been conflicting estimates of casualties at all stages of all wars. However, since the Second World War, few men have remained untraced forever, a change attributed to a policy of 'we will not leave our mates – dead or alive'.

Gallipoli was a prime example of how difficult it can be to properly identify what happened to a casualty and how. Controversial statistics suggest that Anzac and Turkish dead comprised about 30 per cent of their total casualties. British and French forces, on the other hand, lost only about 10 per cent of their total casualties. On the basis of those rounded figures, the Anzacs and Turks must have had either poorer surgical help, much harder fighting, less reliable records, more risk taking or any combination of these possibilities.

Whatever the reasons, when the Allied numbers are viewed alone, there is overwhelming evidence that the Anzacs fared least well of all participants.

FROM SHADOWS ...

Some statistics suggest that about fifteen of every 1,000 Coalition troops serving in Iraq have committed suicide. Separately, 20 per cent of those returning home have some level of clinical anxiety, depression or other stress disorder – about twice as often as might be expected in a similar civilian population. Why mental problems are fewer in soldiers serving in Afghanistan than in Iraq is an unanswered question for investigation. Some sufferers from 'combat stress' who get early intensive therapy have either returned to full duty or remained capable of some other form of service activity. Sustained and complete recovery seems rare, even with protracted, personalised programmes of 'psychological engineering' carried out remotely from conflict.

Counting casualties comes under its greatest scrutiny when it is reported that more than one-quarter of all military deaths occur from 'non-hostile' causes called 'accidents'. Among the victims are 'civilian security men', 'mercenaries' and 'contractors', some of whom habitually resist any precise identification. These 'soldiers of fortune' or 'dogs of war' might fight for anyone anywhere and do almost anything for a large enough fee. Many will fight for any country or its opponent with no sense of loyalty to either. A few are employed simply because of their mastery of particular weapons or tactics and a willingness to accept almost prohibitive risks.

Inevitably, no estimate of the total number of casualties occurring in those individuals can ever be precise when their lives are so cloaked in mystery. Even when badly wounded, many are reluctant to be treated in conventional military hospitals even though they have access to them at no cost. As many are under assumed names it is often impossible to precisely identify them when they die.

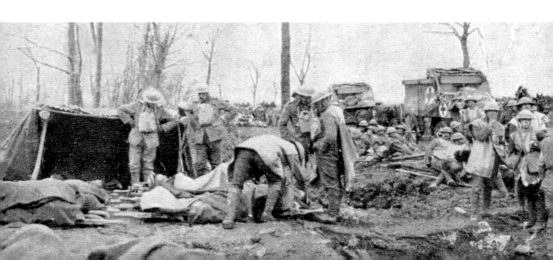

... INTO SUNSHINE

The awful statistics of war divert our attention too easily from less sombre events. The poem 'In Flanders Fields' was the inspiration for the wearing of poppies as a tribute to the men and women who fell in the First World War. Although based on a sad personal loss in a tragic campaign, that enduring, upbeat poem of war was written by Dr John McCrae, a Canadian Army surgeon during the terrible battle of Ypres in the spring of 1915. He wrote it in a field ambulance as he looked out over the endless rows of makeshift graves of his patients. He had already served in the Boer War, but had never become adjusted to the magnitude of the suffering and death that he witnessed on the battlefields of Flanders in Belgium.

After seventeen days of treating terrible injuries, one death particularly affected McCrae. A young friend and former student, Alexis Helmer, was killed before his eyes by a shell. In modern parlance, the boy was almost 'disappeared' by the blast and his remains were scattered widely. What could be found was collected in a sandbag and wrapped in an army blanket closed with safety pins for burial. In the absence of a chaplain, McCrae performed the funeral service, using his prayer book in almost total darkness on the same evening.

While waiting for ambulances to deliver another load of wounded men to his dressing station on the next day, he listened to the larks singing among the shell bursts and admired the wild poppies springing from the soil of the fresh graves before him. The poem was said to be a faithful description of the scene he observed – red poppies swaying gently in the warm wind of a spring morning. But the poem was somewhat more than a word picture. McCrae's last verse was a call for vengeance – to carry on the conflict and win.

> In Flanders Fields the poppies blow
> Between the crosses, row on row,
> That mark our place; and in the sky

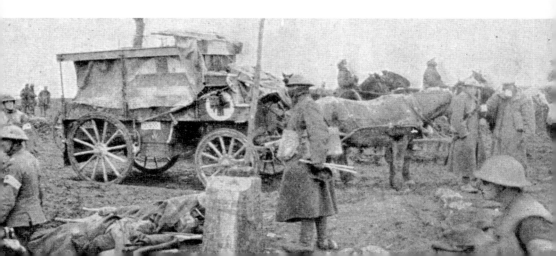

> The larks, still bravely singing, fly
> Scarce heard amid the guns below.
>
> We are the Dead. Short days ago
> We lived, felt dawn, saw sunset glow,
> Loved, and were loved, and now we lie
> In Flanders Fields.
>
> Take up our quarrel with the foe.
> To you from failing hands we throw
> The torch; be yours to hold it high.
> If ye break faith with who die
> We shall not sleep, though poppies grow
> In Flanders Fields.

The poem was published in *Punch* on 8 December 1915 and later reprinted by the *American Ladies' Home Journal* in 1918. It so captivated Moina Michael that she bought hundreds of red paper poppies in memory of the fallen and handed them out to delegates at a conference in New York. McCrae never lived to see the poppies of his poem that have been worn by millions ever since. He probably died of meningococcal septicaemia on 28 January 1918 and was buried where he never wished to be – in the damp earth of Flanders from which poppies rise every year.

More than 5,000 wreaths are donated every Christmas by a local American company to decorate the simple headstones above those lying in the Arlington Military Cemetery in America. With each wreath there is a card carrying a verse that might have pleased McCrae:

> Rest easy, sleep well my brothers.
> Now the line has held, your job is done.
> Rest easy, sleep well.
> Others have taken up where you fell, the line has held.
> Peace, peace, and farewell.

WHITHER IRAQ'S HEALTH?

In 1991, Vern Liebl, an American intelligence specialist during the Gulf crisis, recorded the views of a captured Iraqi officer who had commanded an artillery battalion during Desert Storm. They suggest that, hidden within a belief in 'jihad', is recognition that Allied military and medical teams continue to deliver what is, perhaps, the only tangible form of assistance for all those wounded in current wars. Moreover, help is available from the moment of injury, right up to the Islamic 'gates of paradise' or when they are returned to life. One Iraqi soldier spoke frankly about life under the Hussein regime:

> We are very afraid of Saddam Hussein ... he has spies everywhere ... if I say bad things about him to you, he will kill my wife, my children and my parents ... [he] ... is crazy and there can never be peace if he is alive ... now we have war against the whole world, not just the United States. There were no tactics [used against the Americans] ... we are not logical ... we do not plan ... we do not train ... they just told us to shoot to the last bullet and the last man. Every Iraqi knows that [fighting] is wrong ... I don't wish to go back to Iraq [if Saddam Hussein is President] ... I would rather live in the United States where there is freedom and peace ... the Iraqis are animals with no order or discipline ... every Iraqi is just out for himself.

Just as in Allied forces, Iraqi survivors carry greater physical disabilities than ever before. This Iraqi officer did not seem intent on immediate salvation by self-sacrifice. A perennial issue in the concept of 'shooting to the last bullet and the last man' is what to do when that philosophy leaves a survivor with insufficient residual function to allow a comfortable life. That question has become a matter of profound ethical, moral, practical and community relevance for both sides.

Media headlines are saturated by images of the carnage generated by those who are intent on grabbing what they can get before order is fully restored, at least by Iraqi standards. Sir John Keegan foresees the replacement of Saddam Hussein's regime by small, irresponsible local minorities, all attempting to entrench themselves soundly before some sort of peaceful democracy can develop.

Now that Saddam has gone and the Coalition is re-evaluating its position, a high priority will be given to the maintenance of some sort of sophisticated medical and surgical resources in Iraq and other areas of conflict when Allied combat forces are finally withdrawn. For nearly five years, those services have been available to all indigenous and imported civilians and combatants in Iraq, regardless of their motives and allegiance and gratitude. How much those services will suffer with the process of disengagement remains to be seen. It is predictable that Iraq, and Afghanistan later, will lose a great deal of the medical technology and expertise that they have come to expect, if and when allied military hospitals are decommissioned and expensive resources placed elsewhere. That is the price to be paid for 'independence' and self-reliance.

Illustrations on p. 230–31: scene at an advanced dressing station during a battle, France, First World War.

CHAPTER 18

The Thieves of Minds and Men

The beauty of the world has two edges, one of laughter, one of anguish, cutting the heart asunder.

– Virginia Woolf, *A Room of One's Own*, 1929

The language of war is usually designed to obscure the reality of deliberate and professional mass murder. There is nothing 'casual' about casualties. Basically, the losses of personnel on land, sea or in the air arises not only from combat but also from disease, desertion, capture or accident. With the advent of heavy artillery on the Western Front in the First World War, many of the 'disappeared and missing in action' were stranded on a razed moonscape of shell holes, corpses, water and mud on desolate battlefields from which they could never be retrieved.

Although only a few thousand troops have been actively treated for all grades of structural head or brain injury from service in Iraq (the majority from IED blasts), there may be many others who have not yet sought treatment for commonplace symptoms such as depression, irritability and lost concentration – or those who are yet to manifest any symptoms at all. Obviously, to define a 'significant' head injury as 'one which needs the air-lifting of a man to a military hospital' is misleading – how misleading, remains to be seen.

On the other hand, to include persisting symptoms such as insomnia and ill-defined aches and pains in the category of service-related 'brain injury', when they may be caused by hot weather, heavy duties, civilian-type motor vehicle accidents, sporting activities or simple infections, seems equally inappropriate. Doctors are supposed to avoid concluding that the concurrence of two events necessarily makes them causally related.

Regardless of an army policy of actively seeking evidence of structural brain damage, only a third of troops eligible for veterans' health care have taken it up, despite strong encouragement to do so. Most of their stress symptoms seem to have responded reasonably well to 'three hots and a cot' (three hot meals a day and a bed). Not surprisingly, the closer it looks, the more often the US Army finds problems that might well be attributable to war service.

In older wars, one in every six demobilised troops had some evidence of brain injury, though often ill-defined. Lately, one small experience has suggested that more than one-half of all retired troops have enough 'wrong with their brains' for it to constitute a new syndrome whose criteria and precise causes may never be defined. Happily, the majority of all those not seriously 'addled' by head injury do survive and return to productive military or civilian employment.

SHELL-SHOCK

There are those 'who were there' and survived it all, but whose minds have become haunted by endless shadows. Just as with many of the statistics of war, the most reliable information about casualties comes from doctors and the military hospitals that treat soldiers. Men's complaints are not always physically explicable, but in compiling casualty lists a compromise must be reached to establish the most appropriate category into which a troubled survivor might be placed. Swiss doctors used the poignant term 'nostalgia' for mental disturbance resulting from combat and fear, with its yearning for past circumstances such as home and family and silence. Sufferers displayed symptoms that were atypical, but strangely stereotyped and even ethereal. They often resisted classification and failed to respond to conventional medical or even surgical procedures. Their symptoms could recur and proliferate in unpredictable ways.

Not surprisingly, military surgeons have always been reluctant to become involved in the management of symptoms masquerading, sometimes very convincingly, as physical disorders but lacking common, appropriate and specific diagnostic features. Ultimately, many of the complaints from those patients came to be labelled 'functional' by surgeons and psychiatrists, for want of a better understanding.

'Shell-shock' was the usual Allied Second World War term for the Swiss nostalgia and it was theorised that the unrelenting concussion of heads by explosions could permanently damage brains in some way. The provocative concept of 'the lonely battlefield' was based on the remoteness of bombarding weapons so that all that men could comprehend was the enormous danger from invisible guns firing from somewhere or other unknown to them – perhaps 30 miles away. Instead of getting medical help early in that war, demoralised British soldiers were often executed or imprisoned for cowardice.

One problem in understanding the syndrome was that not all men close to the shells got it, while others far distant from them did. It took a few years of war before the British Army decided that it was often completely impossible to differentiate a shirker or a coward from a good soldier with shell-shock. Before long, the death penalty for cowardice was abolished generally, even by the British.

That came about largely because the task of deciding the issue had been thrust on unwilling medical staff who did not want the responsibility. But even having the death sentence commuted to imprisonment was a terrible and permanent stain on a man's war record.

The widely publicised and supposedly diagnostic 'thousand-yards-stare' of the shell-shocked seemed to be illustrated in photographs of troops in or around action. It was as if they were seeing and hearing things that others were not able to and it wasn't always a troubled stare. Some seemed more perplexed than fearful, almost as if they were the victims of a sick joke. It was first apparent in the trenches of the Western Front in Europe and later in the Second World War in Italy, where torment had become ingrained and escape was impossible.

The French, Germans and Belgians had their own terms for shell-shock, but they all described the same condition. In some Second World War campaigns, Allied military doctors were directed to forget the term 'shell-shock' altogether and instead call the condition 'Not Yet Diagnosed Nervousness' (NYDN). It affected 10 per cent of British officers at some time and about half that number of other ranks who were thought to be less anxious than their officers, whose greater responsibilities led to a greater sense of failure.

By 1916, nearly half of all casualties in all fighting zones had some degree of shell-shock. About 250,000 men were ultimately discharged from the British Army with that diagnosis. Doctors in combat areas, however, were faced with an offensive choice: they were encouraged by military commanders to accept without question that unexplained symptoms were actually cowardice. For that, even with the death penalty removed, harsh discipline and an immediate return to combat were recommended. When that happened, recurrent breakdown was so common that most doctors took the easy route of letting men pass out of combat. Doctors were realising that NYDN soldiers were simply demonstrating the natural biological variations between courage and resilience and resignation to a sense of 'unfairness' and extreme danger that faced them.

In memoirs of his surgical experiences in France in 1918, Dr F. O. Taylor graphically described conditions that, if prolonged beyond a certain variable point, would lead inevitably to 'shell-shock':

There came an indescribable explosion ... the most horrific, though not the loudest, perhaps, that I had ever heard, followed immediately by dull thuds and the sickening sight of men falling, groaning, spouting blood, whole limbs severed, horses frantically breaking loose ... two more explosions followed ... the hut seemed full of frightfully wounded men ... I saw two men die in front of my eyes ... things outside were still appallingly confused ... 50 non-combatants were dead, dying or wounded ... one face haunts me to this day: a fine young American medical officer lay in the hut at the foot of the road, his expression the most horrible and soul-searing I ever saw [with both thighs fractured] ... he was praying for morphia to ease his agony ... the strain of helplessly watching someone suffering while waiting for dressings

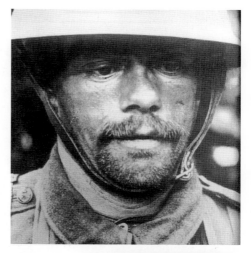

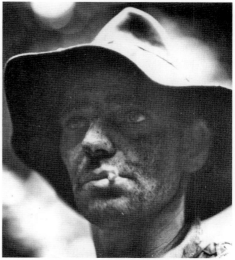

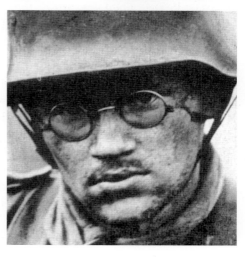

Men of the First and Second World Wars appearing to exhibit exhaustion and probable shell-shock with the so-called 'thousand-yards-stare'.

and drugs to be unpacked [was] insupportable ... my memory here is blurred ... I found a nursing sister [who] had reached the limit of regret ... several hundred stretcher cases still had their first field dressings on ... a beautiful chestnut mare stood patiently tethered to a tree, bleeding slowly to death from a small wound in her belly ... as I had once been a combatant officer, I was beseeched to put an end to her misery with a rifle which was produced from somewhere. All that I can say about this is that I did it ... but it is another haunting memory ... then followed the burial of 29 officers and men ... the service and filling in of the grave took a couple of hours more ... then, in darkness, there were 12 miles to march with exhausted men ... whipping in stragglers ... while cursing them for their bad discipline ... [and tried] ... to be cheerful when we were all in the darkest depths.

In fact, Taylor wondered why all soldiers didn't have shell-shock. Psychiatrists were tossing up theories about that, but in one form or another psychoanalysis and cognitive therapy became the mainstays of management. The results were rarely more than partially and briefly successful. The same disappointment still applies to many cases of civilian 'Post-Traumatic Stress Disorder' (PTSD), which may have no physical fear component in causation. Financial recognition and other compensations are as likely to help as any psychological measures. In war, unless an affected soldier can be physically removed from the source of his intolerable fear, there is little hope of significant recovery.

The Australian ABC programme *Online* ran a story in August 2006 about the British government's posthumous pardoning of more than 300 soldiers who had been executed during the First World War for various reasons. It had become a *cause célèbre* to restore their reputations as worthwhile soldiers. Eighteen of them had been shot for cowardice and most of the others for desertion. These were decisions taken in the heat of battle when the commanders' primary duty was to keep an army fighting and the doctors' duty was to be fully occupied in managing obvious physical injuries. Recently, it has been suggested that these British soldiers were suffering from shell-shock rather than cowardice.

While a complete answer can never be known in particular cases of so long ago, one victim of perfunctory execution was Private Harry Farr who had been hospitalised for five months in 1915 with a diagnosis of shell-shock before returning to his battalion for normal duties on the Somme. After another year of combat, he was in hospital again with the same diagnosis. Shortly after, he was subjected to a twenty-minute court martial for 'cowardice'. Medical evidence in his favour was apparently ignored because no physical disorder had been found. Accordingly, he was shot at dawn next morning. Like some others, he refused a blindfold and faced his firing squad open-eyed.

That type of execution resonates with the fact that eight of the 1,354 Victoria Crosses ever awarded were forfeited (the last in 1908) for offences such as theft of a cow, bigamy and various forms of 'infamous conduct' – entirely out of character with the heroic behaviour that led to a man's decoration. So anomalous were some cases that, in 1920, King George V took a firm hand:

> No matter what the crime committed by anyone on whom the VC has been conferred, the decoration should not be forfeited. Even were a VC [recipient] to be sentenced to be hanged for murder, he should be allowed to wear his VC on the scaffold.

Many troops in the Pacific campaigns of the Second World War complained of 'phantom' symptoms that suggested a surgical condition when investigations failed to identify a physical disorder. Others who had been treated for 'real' abnormalities were slow to recover or never recovered at all, even after surgery performed on reasonable suspicion of a physical disorder.

They had become 'incurable' sufferers from no identified organic abnormality. Faced with increasing numbers of these problems by the end of 1944, the US Surgeon General, Norman T. Kirk, felt obliged to distribute notes on 'The Prevention of Manpower Loss from Psychiatric Disorders'.

For the combat doctor or surgeon so instructed, a heavy, unpleasant responsibility had been conceived. He was expected to treat wounds and illnesses, get men back on duty as soon as possible to forestall the notion of psychiatric disturbance as a satisfactory explanation of continuing symptoms and to shun the use of medical channels to evacuate men who were not sick, just 'non-effective' as the General regarded them.

Evacuating a man from battle on medical grounds had always been the honourable means of sparing him further combat, but commanders did not always agree. General Kirk saw such men as 'goldbricks, cowards and poorly motivated solders [trying to] escape through this channel'. By removing the truly shell-shocked, the General thought the morale of an entire unit might be raised before others were encouraged to find 'occult' reasons to break down. In effect, combat doctors were (quite illogically) left with the ultimate responsibility for deciding if a man's claims were real or false, according to their physical credibility. Once a label of 'shell-shock' had been attached to a soldier, his later physical complaints were usually regarded as pretence. The question then became, 'Should he ever be submitted to combat danger again?' Regardless of the permanently pejorative mark on a man's record, the easy answer was 'no'.

The US Army Surgeon General had anticipated intuitively, and correctly, that there would be worse psychiatric problems after the cessation of hostilities in Europe. Thinking their war was over, many long-serving troops were transferred to the Pacific area and exposed to even more stress. Using statistics, he had calculated that men would break down sooner or later according to a simple mathematical formula: intensity of fear multiplied by its duration. The imponderable factor was 'intensity'. It was certainly the determining factor, but it couldn't be measured as it affected a particular man. On the other hand, 'duration' was easy to calculate.

Infantrymen were by far the most vulnerable to crippling fear, as Surgeon General Kirk recorded:

> Just as an average truck wears out after a certain number of miles, it appeared that the dough boy wore out, either developing an acute incapacitating neurosis, or else becoming hyper-sensitive to shell fire, so overly cautious and jittery that he was ineffective and demoralising to the newer men. The average point at which this occurred appears to have been in the region of 200 to 240 regimental combat days.

Men still on duty after that time had little or no value to their units, but, to complicate that view, the infantryman felt victimised, demoralised and exhausted by prolonged, heavy-combat duties. He was the one at greatest risk but was expected to remain in combat until he had become worthless – 'worn out like a truck'. The army relied on teamwork and pride to keep him going, even as he became more disabled psychologically. Sooner than later, he was easily persuaded by some symptom or event that he was ill and unable to go on. For him, a wound or illness was an undisguised blessing.

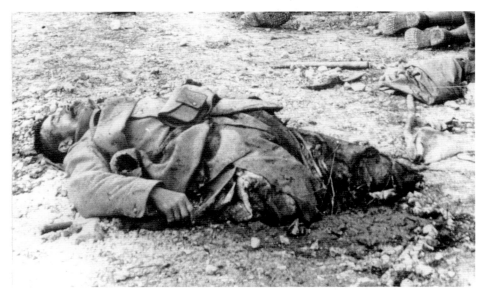

Appalling scenes such as this destroyed all usual senses of value and reality.
(*R. Ruggenberg*)

To extend the dough boys' effectiveness, it was decided that no infantryman should have more than 240 aggregate days of combat before being relieved for at least six months, ideally at home. That policy was applied only to enlisted men in rifle battalions because theirs were the worst jobs in the army. They were to be given priorities in medical care, privileges, provisions, equipment and recreational facilities – all with a heavy accent on being 'respected'. By way of controlling envy, those from other units who might complain about the dough boys' special conditions risked an automatic transfer to the infantry.

However, psychiatrists continued to believe – with little or no possible justification – that any soldier would get better if he could clearly understand the penalties of a lost battle, the strategic significance of his duties, the excellence of his surgical and medical care, and the value of his personal contribution to a foreseeable and successful end to the war. Regardless of those assurances, the use of atomic bombs on Japan was probably brought forward in order to relieve the intolerable burdens of fear and exhaustion in the Allied Pacific forces. Hundreds of thousands of infantry casualties were expected if the Japanese islands had to be invaded and captured.

Inevitably, there is reason to believe that similar stress syndromes are prevalent among troops presently serving in Iraq and elsewhere. Vaccinations for anthrax, plague and whooping cough, and exposure to chemicals used to neutralise nerve agents are increasingly suspected of contributing to stress symptoms and other illnesses.

Time alone will resolve those issues but, in what now seems to have been an absurd verbal flourish, Allied psychiatrists in the Second World War offered an all-purpose solution to men's problems:

> The necessity for mental hygiene ... should be appreciated ... all commanders [should be indoctrinated] with the absolute necessity for a healthy mental outlook in their personnel. In this respect the unit psychiatrist should stand ready to teach the basic principals of mental hygiene and to counsel and advise those requiring this technical equipment.

During the Korean War, an American soldier was twice as likely to become a psychiatric casualty as he was to be killed. After the Vietnam War, more than a million veterans (with varied service experiences) were diagnosed as having PTSD for which there was no entirely satisfactory explanation. Inevitably, there was a perception that some were 'faking it', cowardly, or so weak as to lose their ability to deal with stress altogether. Although disabling shell-shock has not often been documented in medical groups, many doctors were similarly exposed to stress and must have suffered from it and recognised its effects but rarely declared themselves.

An Australian doctor, Griffith Spragg, served as an infantryman in Syria and on the Kokoda Trail before he studied medicine and became a chief adviser in psychiatry to the Department of Veterans' Affairs. In 1970, he worked in a field hospital in Vietnam where he could observe the responses of men under profound stress, as he had in combat. Spragg concluded that the habit of rapidly returning troops with 'war neurosis' to service was inappropriate and often disastrous. He believed that what was called 'combat fatigue' often led to greater psychological disturbance later, whether or not it was then called 'Delayed Stress Reaction', an equivalent of the later 'PTSD'. Spragg's studies of the 'Agent Orange' (AO) issue in Australia and in the USA made him very sceptical of the supposed association between exposure to that chemical and later stress disorders. He was particularly critical of a concentration of attention on financial compensation for exposure when he believed that a more important need was for research into therapy for conventional stress reactions. In 1983, he reported on the urgent need to reassure soldiers in the face of little hard clinical or scientific evidence of AO damage at that time.

He saw a more alarming reaction in some members of the psychiatric staff who regarded veterans' complaints as malingering or exploitation of the issue when there was little correlation between symptoms and exposure levels. Spragg believed that sufferers were genuinely fearful, but would respond to reasonable explanation if it came from objective and temperate professionals. That attitude now seems simplistic and needs a major review with the advantage of better evidence.

Dr Marshall Barr, an anaesthetist who served in Vietnam, has described the effects of war on young medics and operating theatre technicians who were subjected to a variety of traumatic events for which they were not prepared. He regrets that he had overlooked their vulnerability when he accepted their apparent equanimity without question, but his matured perceptions are disturbing:

Counselling has become a trendy, over-used business with professionals creating jobs for themselves and busy-body amateurs taking the opportunity to impart their own prejudiced opinions. In 1967 ... the boys would have laughed at some tame psychologist trying to explore their emotions ... the best I ever offered [the medics and technicians] was the superficial jokiness we shared together when the times were good ... the awful truth ... is that they were affected by their experiences, some very badly. They had seen men of their own age with limbs blown off and bodies ripped by shrapnel. They had taken part in desperate surgical battles with bellies full of blood. They had been handed amputated limbs to be burned. Occasionally they had seen death. The ghastliness was worst when the injuries were caused by accidents with their own [anti-personnel] mines or by 'friendly fire'.

In retrospect it is astonishing that nobody broke down and that the work ... rarely faltered. But the memories were being stored up ... when they got home [they] were subjected to years of abuse and vilification for having served their own country. I was lucky. I had my privileged officer's war [and] then an escape from the national hostility [against the Vietnam veterans]. My psychological traumas were short-lived ... or perhaps not ... I [still] have nightmares flashing back 30 years – terrifying scenes of soldiers horrifically injured and me unable to cope.

In 1990, an unusually demoralising war 'syndrome' arose in Rwanda when troops had to stand by (as ordered by the United Nations) and watch civilians being massacred. Of course, surviving villagers were severely traumatised but counselling is not a service provided in that country. (If a tree falls in that psychological context where there is no one to hear it, there is certainly no sound.) The syndrome affected surgical teams as much as civilians. Medical services in Rwanda were employed as much for peacekeeping and civilian maintenance as they were for combat injuries.

However, wounds were different from those of earlier wars. While trauma from mines had always been common, the average age of the civilian injured in Rwanda was below twenty-five years for the first time. There was a strong suspicion that children were being targeted deliberately. Below-knee amputation became such a common operation that, in one centre, a general surgeon and an orthopaedic surgeon performed 168 amputations in a six-week period. Many injuries in the 'irresponsible', younger community were supposedly caused by undocumented motor vehicle accidents. So extreme were the medical challenges of the region that, at the end of one round of duty, an exhausted surgeon observed, 'There is no surgical training in any country, even in the third world, that can completely prepare a surgeon for conditions such as Rwanda.'

The same could probably apply to all war zones at some time. Surgical teams that witness vast amounts of human destruction daily become susceptible to a sense of revulsion and futility about what they are doing. While that is relieved by the ever-increasing salvage of even the most tragically wounded, survival comes at the enormous cost of permanent disability.

In marked contrast, surgical team members have sometimes developed a very different 'counter-disaster syndrome' – a disturbing belief that they are indispensable or indestructible. That misconception sometimes leads to 'compassion fatigue', which has been described particularly in younger surgeons who are suddenly immersed in intensive, traumatic environments, especially when isolated from senior colleagues. They were considered to be losing compassion, rather than their enthusiasm and competence. There was no panic, desertion or negligence and the outlook was increasingly favourable as their experience grew and their isolation decreased.

In my own fifty years of involvement in various forms of civilian surgery – much of it at the frontiers of difficulty and peril where outcomes were often doubtful and success was sometimes miraculous – I can recall no significant or sustained breakdown in motivated doctors or nurses. In contrast, Dr Michael E. DeBakey, of Baylor College of Medicine in Houston, Texas, wrote in 2007 that this was not uncommon in intensive combat zones of the Second World War. His view was that the most valuable formula for maintaining morale was the unquestioned authority of strong command figures who maintained composure and perspective, whatever the temptations to submit to despair.

Shortly after the Normandy landing in the Second World War, a large number of American anaesthetists beyond the age of forty withdrew from the worst areas and left younger, less-experienced anaesthetists to carry on the complex burdens of the war. Predictably, the response of the surgical and nursing teams was dismay, but it seems that nobody labelled the anaesthetists as weak, shirkers, cowards or disloyal, even though their behaviour constituted desertion on the basis of stress. There are no published studies analysing symptom outcomes in those officers, but some described sensations of 'everything going wrong' so that, years later, even fireworks would evoke inordinate fear and a wish to run away from them.

One observation that often applies to medical personnel at risk of depression is that to achieve one unexpected, vital success in the face of dire jeopardy can invigorate a team more than a dozen 'anticipated wins'.

CHAPTER 19

Bombs, Booby Traps and Land Mines

'Guerrillas' [Spanish for 'little wars'] are irregular troops fighting within areas occupied by the enemy. When they obey the laws of conventional warfare, they are entitled, if captured, to be treated as ordinary prisoners of war but they are often executed by their captors ...

The tactics of guerrilla warfare stress deception and ambush instead of mass confrontation and succeed best in rugged terrain with a sympathetic populace whom guerrillas often seek to win over by propaganda, reform and terrorism.

– Columbia Encyclopaedia, Edition 6, 2008

In its implements and methods, guerrilla warfare is the reverse of 'regular' warfare, but the wounds produced are no different. It consists of small-scale operations spread over an indefinite period. Psychologically, it has been likened to 'fleas biting a dog to death'. The guerrillas' primary intention may or may not be to commit suicide. For the most extreme, it is to kill or maim as many as possible of any age and either sex. If that includes the guerrilla, it is of little consequence to him, her or their families, apart from the automatic acquisition of martyrdom and accelerated salvation. For others, such as the European 'underground' movements of the Second World War, activities were directed primarily at sabotaging the occupying forces' means of making war. To say the least, to lose life in underground combat represented a serious failure and waste of personnel.

Suicide bombers usually carry their equipment in their clothing in order to be sure of when and where the explosion will occur from self-activation or from a remote source. Alternatively, bombing may be carried out from cars, trucks or aeroplanes and may not necessarily involve suicide. Commonly, a bomb-loaded vehicle is abandoned and detonated by distant command. However it is done, the damaging effects on humans are a source of surgical horror. In the interests of survival of those at risk from suspected suicide bombers, an urgent, violent response to suspected danger is essential, ideally from a supposedly protected position.

Booby traps and improvised explosive devices (IED) come in all sizes, shapes and designs, with an array of methods of placement. Components usually come from defence-force stocks and commercial hardware stores, or from international black markets. Their effects are limited only by the ingenuity of the bomber. Their casualties and terror can accomplish powerful tactical goals, the net effect of which is a pervading suspicion of all unusual objects and movements, a constant strain on morale and such a level of fear that all purposeful mobility is inhibited.

When devices are grouped or inter-connected, the heart-breaking multiplicity of wounds is further magnified. Measures proven to increase survival include the wearing of protective clothing, sandbagging the floors of vulnerable vehicles, opening windows or hatches to reduce effects of concussive blast and discouraging public transport travel generally – particularly passengers standing in buses and trains.

Land mines are attractive to lone insurgents because they are cheap, small, easy to manufacture and position, and can provide a major obstacle to terrestrial military action. They are exploded by remote electronic triggering, sound, trip-wire, wireless, radio, telephone or by the pressure of a foot or vehicle. The overall ambition of those who sow mines is probably to wound rather than kill, because injured survivors consume disproportionate amounts of evacuation, and surgical and supportive resources. Mines accounted for 50 per cent of all injuries treated by Soviet surgeons in the Afghanistan War of 1979–89. Many of them were manufactured and planted by Russians before they were dug up and used by the Afghans. To complicate 'inter-personal' matters further, the Americans also supplied the Afghan tribesmen with weapons to fight the Russian invaders.

Blast and shrapnel at ground level cause catastrophic injuries to the legs and lower body. The Russians in Afghanistan found that many casualties required huge blood transfusions for resuscitation – much larger than previously used for similar injuries. Blast injuries of the heart, lungs, brain, spinal cord and all gas-containing organs carried a high mortality and most limb injuries were multiple, many of them requiring immediate amputation. Overall, the Russian understanding was that, 'good judgement comes from experience and experience comes from poor judgement'.

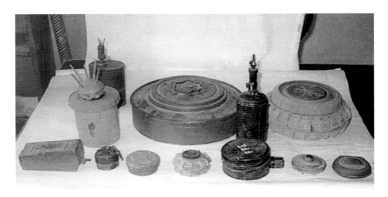

Land mines for various anti-personnel or anti-vehicle purposes, according to size, distance, position and vulnerability of targets. (*Wikipedia*)

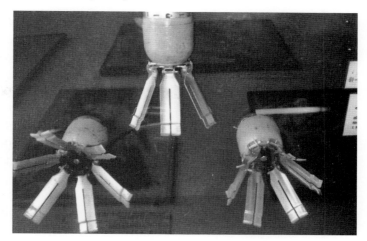

Russian parachute mines employed in Vietnam, designed to drop slowly enough to reach the ground before detonation. (*Saigon War Museum*)

CHILDREN IN WAR

Landmines represent the most toxic pollution facing mankind.

– International Committee of the Red Cross, 1994

Every year, surgeons are called on to mend the mine-shattered bodies of more than 10,000 children somewhere in the world. In Red Cross units in Afghanistan, Cambodia, Somalia and Rwanda, 50 per cent of all landmine victims are children. Cambodia still contains twice as many landmines as children. Because of their small size and innate curiosity, children are more likely than adults to be severely injured or killed. Large numbers of them lose more than one limb and have devastating injuries to their trunks, genitals and faces. Blinding is common.

As a result, many children never attend school or have relationships because of their disabilities or disfigurement. They might wait ten years to obtain a prosthetic limb and then, with body growth, their prostheses would normally need to be changed every few years, but that is impossible in such poor countries.

It is widely rumoured that during the Iran–Iraq war of the 1980s, children were used as minefield sweepers before danger areas were entered by the military. Small and doomed groups of children less than ten years of age were sent out to act as 'human waves' and risk mutilation. Guerrilla groups in Central Africa have been accused of employing children for spying and reconnaissance in areas where an enemy scarcely notices them. Some are programmed to plant small mines as they roam among unsuspecting communities. 'Boy soldiers' seem to be widely used.

Inevitably, undiscovered mines prohibit entry to affected areas to the extent that free movement, commerce and agriculture cannot continue. Because it may take years before they can be cleared or exploded, mines set today may still be killing and maiming for decades. One strategy to reduce injuries from concealed mines is to limit travel to places where animals or humans have left recent tracks – safer than making new paths, but even that precaution is never absolutely reliable.

Many mine-victim children survive long enough to be injured more than once because they forget caution in handling unusual objects they find. In Iraq, they have died from using live disc mines as go-cart wheels. The most resourceful manufacturers have devised special features to attract children, such as the Russian 'butterflies' and brightly-coloured objects resembling trinkets, toys and ornaments. Unexploded devices remain in many areas of Iraq, Cambodia, Afghanistan, Columbia, Laos, Vietnam and Angola. In Cambodia, mines are frequently redeployed by families to protect property, settle disputes and blast fish from rivers.

Angola alone has 100,000 mine amputees – 10,000 being children. Frequently, parents are injured in the same explosion, orphaning their children. A bonus for all mine-layers is that their 'baits' act as excellent, economical, surrogate troops. They require no salary or ongoing cost, rarely miss their target and, like other instruments of killing, they are impersonal and soulless. While a mine may cost only a few dollars to manufacture, it might need hundreds of dollars to remove by time-consuming, dangerous and expensive work. Few war-torn nations have the resources to properly mount any effective, removal programme.

A small number of explosive weapons continue to be distributed by air, despite being widely 'banned' by international agreement. The resulting wounds provide crash-courses in trauma surgery for teams working in the 'third world'. Aside from a mine ban being introduced by some nations, it has also been suggested, with little optimism, that those who sell mines should be taxed to fund their later clearance, to educate victimised populations and to rehabilitate and maintain the innocent, lifelong sufferers. Time will tell if that will ever be agreed.

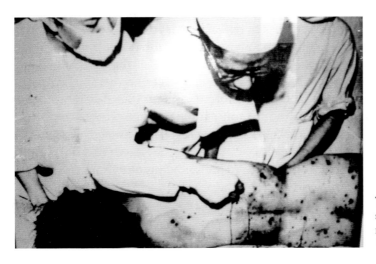

Typical impacted shrapnel wounds of many sizes. (*Saigon War Museum*)

CHAPTER 20

The Arms Merchants

The series of weapons developed by Kalashnikov includes self-loading carbines, sniper rifles, automatic pistols, assault rifles, machineguns and sub-machineguns, magazines for various weapons, with bayonets and knives fitted as optional extras. As a collector's item, a short version of the AK47 is available with a silencer and grenade launcher.

– Kalashnikov assault rifles catalogue, Prospect Books, London, 1955

While the 'laws' of war are concerned with limiting the use of weapons such as landmines, surgical teams that deal with the catastrophic effects of those weapons are at the forefront of efforts to control their indiscriminate sale. Ambitions to make such arms illegal are not altogether hopeless when it is considered that the short sword, the crossbow and longbow, the dum-dum and the French Minié bullets, the machine-gun, and the poison-gas and bio-weapons have each, at some time, been considered sufficiently repugnant to warrant their banning – and some bans have succeeded.

An interest in gas warfare as a weapon of mass destruction goes back centuries. In more recent times during the Iran–Iraq war, both sides were accused of employing chemical and biological weapons; it was estimated that more than 100,000 Iranians were damaged by them. In that prolonged conflict, many companies from many nations (including twenty-four American firms) simultaneously supplied precursors of those devices to both sides.

By any measure, the arms industry is a giant global consortium whose products are aimed to kill and maim people, keeping surgical teams constantly busy worldwide. Various estimates place the annual international expenditure on weapon products at around US$1,000 billion. The countries and international companies that manufacture and sell weapons are well known. Lockheed Martin sold US$34 billion of defence materials to the world in 2004. That constituted almost all of its revenue for that year. Boeing sold US$30.5 billion of similar equipment – more than half of its total revenue. In 2008, Britain became the world's largest arms seller.

Aside from the USA and UK, other less well-known exporting countries listed in 2005 included, in no particular order, the Netherlands, France, Italy, Japan, Sweden, Germany, Israel, Russia, India, Singapore, Spain, South

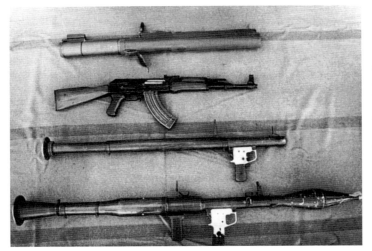

Types of weapons usually employed by third world insurgents or 'freedom-fighters'. An AK47 is second from top and a rocket-propelled grenade launcher bottom. (*Kalashnikov small-arms catalogue, 1955*)

Korea, Australia, Norway, Canada, Brazil and Finland. Cumulatively, their product sales are enormous. Small items available for sale include pistols, shotguns, revolvers and 'other firearms', unspecified 'accessories', ammunition containers, handcuffs, batons, personal rocket launchers, anti-riot equipment and armoured clothing. Anything from a baton to a nuclear weapon can be bought somewhere.

Most industrialised countries have a domestic arms industry for their own use, but also sell to other countries and non-sovereign states – particularly those with political instability. Huge numbers of arms are sold on without trace. Contract verification is obscured by covert links between commercial, military and political beneficiaries. It is disturbing to learn that Russian ground-to-air systems are one of its most exported military products and that India and China were the biggest buyers in 2002 and 2004.

The best-selling, semi-automatic AK47 rifle has been produced in greater numbers than any other weapon in recorded history and has been used in conflicts all over the world for sixty years. Since General Kalashnikov first developed his gun in 1947, there have been many modifications offered by licensed manufacturers in and outside Russia to satisfy the special needs of clients. With little basic training, any child or adult of either sex can learn to deliver the AK47's 650 rounds per minute expertly. Because of its simplicity and reasonable cost, it has been preferred universally by insurgents, often supplied by Communist nations that buy them at bargain-basement prices from major producers and then retail them to third world countries.

Although General Kalashnikov derived little direct wealth from his gun, for which he had no patent, he had no hesitation in promoting a new vodka branded with his name. Unfortunately for him, the word 'Kalashnikov' is already written into history after decades of immeasurable terror and death.

The 'Leahy Law' of 1997 was intended to prevent the export of military products and know-how to countries that had committed human rights abuses. Within that putative limitation, the US Defence Department disposes of articles produced in excess of sales by donation or re-sale at bargain-basement prices to selected buyers for 'education and training'. According to Congress reports, most US arms contracts in 2005 were made with developing countries for 'research and warfare-simulation studies'.

Those sales translate directly to astronomic human devastation somewhere in the world every day. Clearly, there are potent moral issues when profits are allowed to vastly outweigh concepts of peace and the value of lives. Fortunately, some investors are disinclined to become involved overtly in arms sales to violent countries, especially when the marketing of weapons may be a very expensive exercise.

Even more sensitive issues involve the placing of American troops in conflict with other troops who have been trained by their own military and are employing identical weapons. Such issues have an important negative impact on arms exports, which are recognised increasingly as unnecessary, unprincipled and evil.

The International Red Cross reports that half of all war casualties treated in under-privileged countries are civilians caught in crossfire. Much of their and others' medical treatment is provided free or at low cost in state-financed hospitals. At the same time, subsidies for arms exporters in most countries are almost as generous as those for agriculture. After the 'Cold War' wound down two decades ago, arms production declined considerably, only to escalate later in response to the demands of Africa, China and India. It has been estimated that most of today's arms traders sell AK-47s and other weapons freely to places like sub-Saharan Africa, Palestine, Yemen, Sri Lanka, Iran, Iraq, Pakistan and South America, where insurgents such as Al-Qaeda and Hamas control their distribution to hundreds of thousands of child terrorists. Those regimes buy cheap arms from the big players and receive training as part of purchasing contracts.

Aggressively competing suppliers from other nations have begun to challenge the USA for a market share of the arms industry. To its credit, America is said to have ceased exporting ballistic and cruise missiles and anti-personnel landmines. Notions of accountability may one day cause the world to stop and think again. After all, terrorist organisations get their arms from wherever they can and they cannot be banished without developed countries possessing the same sorts of arms, usually derived from the same sources. Therein lies the absurd circuit of destruction that must be broken if wisdom is to prevail.

In the meantime, the deadly products provided by arms factories create human suffering and keep medical teams overwhelmed throughout much of the underprivileged world. Remarkably, most 'developed' countries continue to spend more on military medicine and defence than on civilian health care.

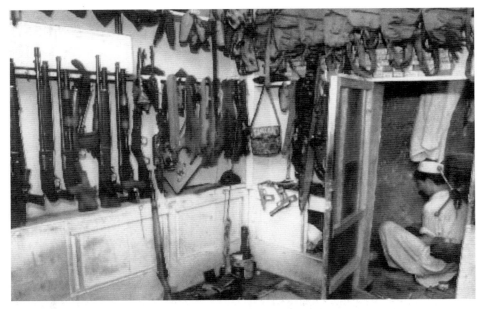

A gunsmith's factory and showroom, Pakistan, 2001. (*IRC*)

The distinguished British medical journal *Lancet* is one of the world's largest and most respected journals. In September 2005, one of its editorials drew attention to the fact that its publisher, Reed Elsevier, was also fostering some of the world's largest arms promotions. The most recent event was a 'Defence Systems and Equipment International' exhibition in London in 2006. *Lancet*'s editors strongly rejected any relationship between the journal and the arms trade and suggested that 'the world's leading medical publisher (Reed Elsevier) should align its business values with the professional values of the majority of those it serves'.

Cluster bombs were freely available at an associated arms fair in 2006, where 60 per cent of sales were to developing countries. Many doctors worldwide complained that Elsevier's involvement in the arms fair was incompatible with *Lancet*'s guiding principles, which include the maxim, 'to do no harm'. In reply to such complaints, Elsevier claimed that the defence industry was 'central to the preservation of freedom and national security. The role of the armed forces now often includes disaster-relief work and humanitarian exercises.'

To that apparent obfuscation, *Lancet*'s editors pointed out that the journal had a long record of drawing attention to the adverse health consequences of war and violence. Therefore, any perceived connection between the journal and the arms trade, 'no matter how tangential it may be', must be rejected completely. After years of such worldwide protests, Elsevier finally listened to his customers, authors and staff, and in June 2007 he agreed to terminate such presentations by the end of that year. No doubt, many eyes will be watching Elsevier's future activities closely.

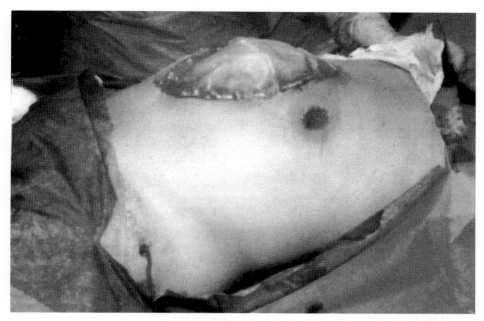

A massive abdominal gunshot injury, Iraq; wound closure has been delayed by a temporary plastic-sheet closure to accommodate swelling; there is a temporary colostomy to the right of the plastic patch. (*Dr G. Peoples*)

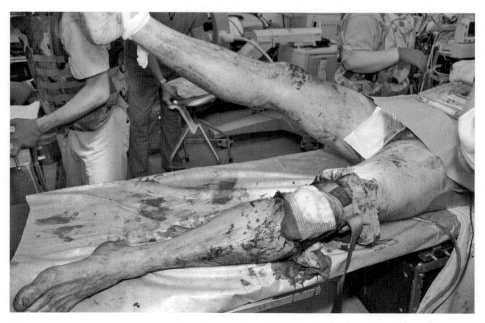

Cluster-bomb damage to an Iraqi civilian in Balad Hospital, Iraq, 2004. (*Dr G. K. Bruce*)

CHAPTER 21

The Faces of Terror

Every man has reminiscences which he would not tell to everyone but only his friends. He has other matters in his mind which he would not reveal even to his friends, but only to himself, and that in secret. But there are other things which a man is afraid to tell even to himself, and every decent man has a number of such things stored away in his mind.

– Fyodor Dostoyevsky, *Notes from Underground*, 1864

'Terrorism' is defined by *The Oxford Companion to Military History* as, 'the deliberate creation and exploitation of fear through violence or its threat'. It generates an abiding fear that becomes a universal disturbance at some community level. Perhaps a concentration on that process and the energy of the modern media have given terrorism an impact out of proportion to the physical damage, but the threat produces a profoundly morbid, psychological effect.

That terrorism pervades the daily life of much of the world's population is not surprising. Anti-terrorist measures have impinged on every facet of some communities – medical, military and police forces, travellers, workers, families, schools and political systems. Mass-transport systems such as airlines, railways and buses are particularly attractive to terrorists, but the most dramatic target of all is an aeroplane filled with passengers.

Since 1983, there have been many opportunistic terrorist bombings: the US embassies in Beirut, Kenya and Tanzania; a Pan-Am flight over Lockerbie; an Air India flight over the Irish Sea; a UTA flight over Chad; the World Trade Centre, New York; the Federal Building, Oklahoma City; a military complex in Saudi Arabia; a Jewish Centre in Buenos Aires; the USS *Cole* in Aden; buses in Colombo and Israel; tourist groups in Egypt; Omagh in Northern Ireland; a Moscow apartment; a discothèque in Tel Aviv; a Bali tourist centre; a Mumbai hotel; and an Islamabad market. Clearly, the possibility of attacks cannot be ignored in any place where politically sensitive targets exist, and so they continue without adequate control.

An aborted 2006 plot to blow up ten airliners simultaneously was the most serious mass threat since the September 2001 aircraft attacks in America. In this case, liquid explosives were to be concealed within sports drink bottles and detonated by disposable-camera flashes. The threatened travellers were predominantly tourists – even if any had survived, no medical resource could have begun to deal with the situation adequately. Twenty-four suspected perpetrators were arrested and found to have their sophisticated suicide operation at an advanced stage of planning. Two of those arrested had already prepared martyrdom tapes. Other members of the team were still being sought in 2007.

In 1995, a similar plan to destroy three airliners every hour for three hours as they crossed the east coast of the USA was described by a US security official as an 'iconic' piece of terrorism. In response, the author John le Carré wrote in *The Times* of London of the worsening catastrophe of terrorism and his own difficulty in responding to it. He viewed terror as a macabre form of theatre:

> Dare I fly? Or am I to tell police about the weird couple upstairs? Would it be safer not to drive down Whitehall this morning? Is my child safely back from school? Have my life savings plummeted?

Long before, in his book *The Secret Pilgrim*, le Carré had written a personal observation of Middle Eastern terrorism, describing the things ambulance crews and surgical teams see every day somewhere. Nothing has changed:

> It was one of those seasons in Beirut when you could set your watch by the first excitements of the evening. But I have never minded too much about the shooting. Shooting has a logic, if a haphazard one. It's directed at you, or away from you. My personal phobia was car bombs – never knowing as you hurried along a pavement or dawdled in the sweaty, crawling traffic, whether a parked car was going to take out an entire block with one huge heave, and leave you in such tiny shreds that there was nothing worth a body bag, let alone a burial. The thing you noticed about car bombs – I mean afterwards – was shoes. People blown clean out of them, but the shoes intact. So that even after the bits of body had been picked out and taken away, there was still the odd pair or two of wearable shoes among the broken glass and smashed false teeth and shreds of someone's suit. A little machinegun fire, like now, or the odd hand-held rocket, didn't trouble me as much as [they did] some people.

While psychologists have examined situations where humanity lives on the verge of catastrophe, they have rarely emphasised the unique roles of medical teams in salvaging something from the frightening uncertainties that terrorism has created. Once diplomacy, reasoning, threats, sanctions and surveillance have failed, there is no practical and available protection apart from a medical one. Inevitably, doctors and nurses and their teams fear and loathe terrorism and guerrilla damage as much as anyone else, but they never expected these forms of conflict to generate a scale of casualties that would dominate their work.

In Almogy and Rivkind's surgical experience of terrorism in Jerusalem in 2005, typical 'triage' meant maximum care for the saveable and no active care for the irreversibly doomed. They recognised that the basic aim of terrorism was to generate fear, confusion, horror, panic and, most importantly, to change people's behaviour in everyday life. They realised that their large trauma centres could just manage fifteen severely injured patients arriving within an hour but, beyond that, ancillary reception centres were urgently needed to expand services.

To achieve maximum devastation, suicide bombers often choose to detonate their equipment in the centre of crowds where even low-grade explosives produce severe injuries by blast waves, collapsed buildings and shrapnel. Victims in confined spaces are always the most damaged.

Like others before them, Almogy and Rivkind saw blast destruction of body organs that contained gas, such as the lungs, bowels and ears, but many victims also had shrapnel and debris injuries and severe burns. One in five survivors had massive, open fractures of more than one limb. This pattern of terror-bombing damage is quite common.

In response, Israeli hospitals have developed a systematic reaction, where the most experienced surgeon available is appointed 'surgeon-in-charge' with no active role in direct patient care. All available medical staff are immediately summoned through public announcements and every volunteer is urgently pressed into service of some sort. Teams are directed to emergency, radiology and triage areas.

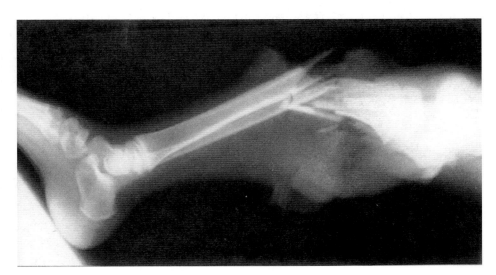

Shattered, unstable, open fracture of tibia and fibula (shin) with marked soft-tissue shredding. The likelihood of damage to large blood vessels makes amputation almost certain.

The injured are sorted and labelled to ensure that those who seem recoverable are treated first. Immediate life-saving procedures are performed at the injury site before transporting victims to special centres in various parts of the city. Those with more than 30 per cent deep burn areas, blown-off limbs and blasted, open fractures usually die at the injury site. They are given the lowest treatment priority, apart from heavy dosage of morphine and comforting. Removal of the dead from areas of injury is deferred until the living have been processed.

The surgeon-in-charge is responsible for repeated triage that must be very pragmatic. Injuries that at first sight might seem manageable may rapidly change to a 'waste-of-time' category. Those with multiple injuries, particularly of the head, chest and abdomen, rarely survive, regardless of the best care. Surgical teams consist of three general surgeons and three anaesthetists in each hospital. Their job is to keep the trauma unit clear of 'minor' cases and to have a rapid turnover of more favourable, though serious, cases.

The Israeli teams believe that the uncertainty and confusion experienced in the Madrid train bombings of 2004 should have been avoidable. Even so, 80 per cent of those admitted to an intensive-care ward in Madrid were thought to require long-term lung ventilation which often led nowhere. That is an

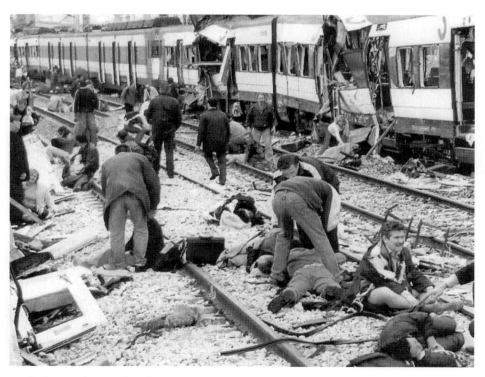

Multiple suicide train bombings in Madrid, 2004, with many dead and injured; confusion and inadequate resuscitation made management almost impossible. (*Santi Acera Tejeda*)

intolerable load to be placed on the resources of most cities. The number of available surgeons, particularly specialists, is usually inadequate when a large group of urgent casualties arrive at once.

To provide additional beds, recovering patients are rapidly transferred out of intensive-care wards to allow for new admissions. Ventilators, pumps and blood are urgently acquired from any available source, including retailers. Efficient rostering by the surgical director is crucial and all available personnel, from interns to heads of departments, are expected to be on active duty whenever required. Retired medical personnel are encouraged to re-enlist for urgent duties.

Staff involved in the profoundly distressing identification and management of severely injured people receive counselling and frequent rotations of duty. Digital photography is used in reception and operative areas while, using mini-cameras on helmets and in ambulances, tele-video contact is maintained between the accident scene, evacuation vehicles and hospitals. To accelerate identification, great care of personal belongings and the establishment of an information centre are fundamental needs.

Many of the lessons coming out of Israel concern civilians who must accept a strict limitation of their numbers on public transport. Standing passengers on buses and trains are warned that they are at much greater risk than when sitting. Higher-backed and cushioned seats in vehicles are being installed to diminish the injury from explosions beneath floors. Those who have access to protective vests are asked to wear them at all times of risk and private travel in suspect areas is severely restricted. All measures require frequent review, rehearsal and dissemination of information in the media.

11 SEPTEMBER 2001

Shortly after the 11 September 2001 aerial attacks on the Twin Towers of the World Trade Center in New York, Amir Moussa, Secretary-General of the Arab League, advised Jeffrey Goldberg of *The New Yorker* (8 October 2001) that, 'All of us will fight terrorism, confront terrorism, but not necessarily by conducting a military campaign.' With US soldiers still in Iraq, Ben Knight of ABC News Online reported (8 December 2009) that violence in Iraq had dropped dramatically with the fewest deaths in November (122) since the US invasion of 2003. The present 115,000 troops are to be reduced to 50,000 in 2010 with complete withdrawal in 2011.

That means that foreign medical and surgical resources, mostly US, will also be reduced or removed, leaving military and predominantly civilian Iraqis without the substantial and sophisticated support provided free and without discrimination since 2003. But Knight also reported that in December 2009, massive car bombings, presumably by Al Qaeda-linked militants, had killed

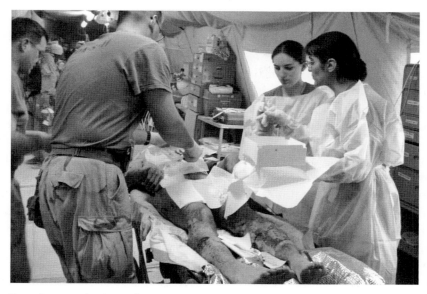

Inserting monitoring tubes into a patient with extensive lower limb injuries caused by a roadside IED, Iraq, 2004; bilateral amputations seem likely. (*Dr G. Peoples*)

127 civilians and wounded another 182. No doubt Iraqis are again asking how they will manage when the great US hospitals are gone and the indigenous people have to fend for themselves without foreign help.

Between 8.46 a.m. and 10.28 a.m. on a balmy weekday autumn morning in 2001, four aerial attacks occurred in north-east America, probably engineered by fifty individuals including nineteen suicidal terrorists. All terrorists and passengers in four high-jacked planes were killed. Whether that constituted a 'war' or a 'crime' is of no consequence. Suddenly, the comfort, confidence, morale, credulity, equanimity and future of the world had been disturbed by highly sophisticated, integrated, lethal vandalism. The damage was inestimable for countless months, and it continues. The demands placed on hospitals, doctors, nurses, police, first-aid staff, fire officers, local port authorities, volunteers, defence forces and general resources were enormous and enduring.

The atmospheric and psychic savagery of the day were shocking beyond all experience, worsened by the ignorance of those who had committed the attacks, raising questions of what it meant, what to do, how to protect oneself and others, how to communicate and what the future held for people and the planet. Nearly 3,000 of 17,000 civilians in the Twin Towers and nearby perished within a few hours, regardless of all available medical and surgical services at several hospitals. Some 200 occupants of the towers jumped to their deaths. The tragedy of Pearl Harbor had suddenly paled into relative insignificance.

The physical damage confronted by untold numbers of selfless rescuers included immediate, untreatable injuries and almost immediate death from crushing, electrocution, burns, gas and smoke inhalation and fractures. But most of all, those reaching local hospitals suffered from unrelenting fear and panic. The number of late deaths and disabilities has yet to be decided but, years later, severe lung and blood disorders and cancers continue to come to notice, presumably from chemical inhalation. Inevitably, the task of managing such unexpected, varied and massive trauma at short notice, and continuing for weeks, months and years, outstripped all local medical and civil resources. Incompetent, overloaded radio and telephonic connections compounded the tasks confronting hospitals and their staffs.

Such was the nature of the attacks that most deaths were early and impossible to treat. Relatively few were treated for significant injuries in hospitals. The closest regional treatment facility, the New York Downtown Hospital, treated 350 walking wounded in the first few hours and another 1,200 patients on the first day. Few needed surgical attention though burns were a significant problem. Bellevue Hospital reported about ninety people attending by 3.30 p.m. on 9/11, but most had only minor physical injuries produced by inhalation and eye injuries from dust and fumes. Only five operations for non-life threatening fractures, burns and blunt trauma were performed within the first five hours of admission to that major facility.

A similar number of attendances occurred on the next day at other local hospitals, all of which experienced damage to communication devices of all types, and water, gas and electrical services. All hospitals instituted systems of rapid emergency services though most were not required. There were many instances of conflicting, confused or redundant command integration, but one observation was universal – the unbelievably selfless and enduring bravery of fire, police, ambulance, first-aid, port authority staff and volunteers.

During the following months and years, several important aspects have become clear. Apart from hospitals put on emergency systems almost immediately, most casualties were fatal and occurred so soon after the attacks that the victims were not amenable to any treatment apart from first aid. Organisational aspects were less than useful, simply because of the frightening, unexpected and sudden nature of massive, inconceivable damage.

Many reviews of these unique events have concluded that unified command and better, ongoing training and equipping of emergency services are essential. Those decisions were put to the test in Hurricane Katrina in New Orleans when more effective command posts were established to communicate and coordinate efforts to eliminate redundant searches for the missing. But overall, it is accepted that a momentous, immediate, preconceived, multicentric attack of this sort, similar to a massive earthquake, tsunami, shipping or aeroplane disaster, poses problems of salvage never before experienced and unlikely to ever be manageable by established medical and surgical services.

CHAPTER 22

Amputees –
The Everlasting Army

A disabled person who fights back is not handicapped – but is inspired. Don't listen to anyone who tells you that you can't do this or that. That's nonsense. Make up your mind [that] you'll never use crutches or a stick, and then have a go at everything.

– Douglas 'Tin legs' Bader, Second World War fighter pilot ace.
The Douglas Bader Foundation, 1982

Ever since organisms have had limbs and appendages, accidental or deliberate amputation of one or more of them has been commonplace. It is believed that amputation was performed nearly 50,000 years ago by surgeons in Peru, Egypt and Greece for punitive, ritualistic or therapeutic reasons. There is also evidence that prosthetic limbs were fitted in those distant centuries.

When performed deliberately for a limb that, in civilian life, is already 'dead, deadly or a dead loss', surgical amputation limits disability and accelerates total recovery, but at the expense of disfigurement and the loss of a major body part. It is a calculated compromise. In war, the surgical amputation of one or more limbs is often essential, but falls predominantly and abruptly on younger men, imposing an unexpected, lifelong restriction. Regardless of the excellence of prostheses, loss of most of an upper limb means a 60 to 70 per cent loss of 'whole-person' capability, while amputation of most of a lower limb carries a 30 to 50 per cent whole-person loss.

Horatio Nelson would not have had his right arm removed without anaesthesia if his injury had occurred fifty years later. If we can believe the reports, 200 men lay awake during one long day at Borodino while Larrey, Napoleon's chief army surgeon, amputated one or more of their limbs. He was rewarded much later for his skill as a military surgeon. He had always yearned to be buried alongside Napoleon at Les Invalides in Paris, but that site had been reserved for more significant persons like governors, marshals and kings. However, in 1992 the French government finally relented, deciding that Larrey's surgical brilliance justified his remains being re-buried in Paris beside his beloved Napoleon.

The advent of general anaesthesia changed the whole history of amputation because great haste to get the painful job done with a wakeful patient was no

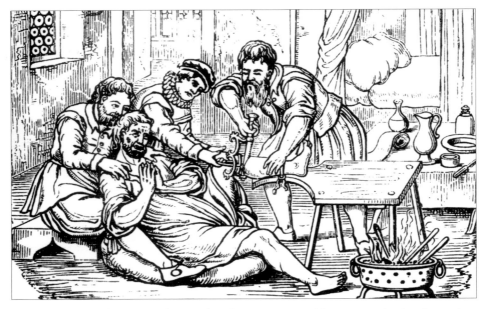

Another graphic depiction of a Medieval amputation without anaesthesia; the patient prays as an assistant tightens a tourniquet and the surgeon's tools are boiled lower right. (*Wikipedia*)

longer required, and a more careful operation was possible. Powerful physical restraint, throttling, biting bullets and intoxication by alcohol or other drugs was no longer necessary by the middle of the nineteenth century. Even the assistance of Dr Joseph Guillotin, who devised the 'guillotine' for the express removal of heads and postulated the value of a similar instrument for limbs, was no longer needed. Surgeons could now take their time with pain-free, sleeping patients. With a developing awareness of antiseptic surgery in the last 120 years, there has been remarkable improvement in the management and recovery rates of amputation performed for any reason.

Amputation became the hallmark of the American Civil War in which more limbs were removed than in any other war in history. It was so common, and often done with such abandon, that two surgeons, Cooper and Stevens, prepared a pocket-sized, 'how-to' manual for inexperienced surgeons to carry in battle areas. It detailed techniques of amputation and stump preparation for prostheses. Their advice to remove 'as little flesh as possible ... and the more bone the better' was accompanied by copious illustrations. Unfortunately, that conservative teaching invited deep infection and gangrene with the likelihood of further amputation.

In war, the surgeon has little control over the length of a stump, but the science of artificial limbs has improved to the point where almost any amputation stump, of whatever length and in whichever limb, can now be fitted with a useful, comfortable and durable prosthesis. Combat injuries tend to be similar to severe civilian trauma, but soft tissue shredding and shrapnel infiltration usually make battle amputations more urgent and often multiple.

Dr Charles Fox of the Walter Reed Army Medical Center reported a greatly increased salvage of limbs threatened by severe damage to blood vessels and haemorrhage simply by improving on the same techniques that have been practiced for decades. That means the urgent application of more effective and less damaging tourniquets, rapid application of special clot-promoting wound dressings and maximum rapid resuscitation from shock by whole blood and clot enhancers. In addition, early opening by 'fasciotomy' of tense, constricting muscle sheaths of swollen limbs and immediate, expert, vascular surgery for reconstruction of arteries by borrowed vein segments or Dacron tubular grafts proved essential.

In major specialist American units, new amputees are rapidly indoctrinated with stories of the accomplishments of other amputees – one-legged Olympic skiers, a double-amputee Everest climber, thousands of Paralympics athletes and the Second World War fighter ace, Sir Douglas Bader, who lost both legs below the knee in an air accident in 1931, but went on to fly again with the RAF. No doubt those examples are inspiring but, as in countless wars before them, the new amputees require enormous rehabilitative assistance and counselling to begin to accept the permanent changes that have happened to their bodies.

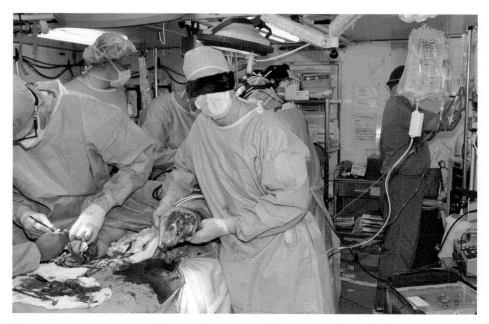

Three surgeons remove two limbs and correct head injuries, Balad, 2008. (*Dr G. K. Bruce*)

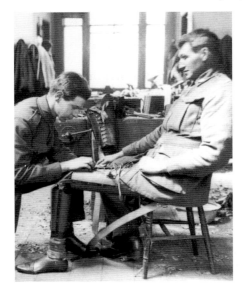
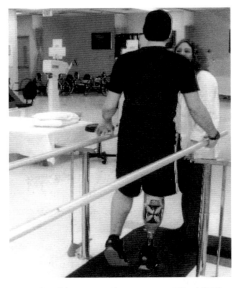

Above left: A French soldier being fitted with an artificial leg (prosthesis), First World War. (*R. Ruggenberg*)

Above right: An Iraqi amputee practises walking on his prosthesis with encouragement from rehabilitation staff. (*Dr G. Peoples*)

ANGELS OF MERCY

The celebrated American Legion Auxiliary Unit 270 has described the humanity displayed at the Walter Reed Army Medical Center (WRAMC), caring for the victims of war. The following comments, based on the personal experiences of two volunteers, are in stark contrast to recent criticisms of standards of care for troops in the WRAMC. It is quite clear that this facility has been heavily overburdened by the challenges of convalescent troops from recent war zones and their entitlement to massive, continuing support:

> You start the day serving breakfast in a dormitory on the camp for 200 wounded soldiers who no longer need the 24-hour care of Walter Reed Army Medical Center Hospital as they are fitted for their prostheses, recover from wounds, and undergo physical therapy.
>
> When the teenage soldier with one arm extends his tray, you thank him for his service to his country and tell him all of America appreciates the sacrifice he has made to protect our freedom.
>
> When a concerned father pushes his son's wheelchair up, you want to say something. You know that the doctors at WRAMC will soon replace the lost legs with state-of-the-art prostheses, but it is still hard to find the right words to express your feelings.

After breakfast you head to the hospital. As you get off the elevator, you see a soldier who lost both arms. You walk up to him and give him a hug. Words are not necessary. He knows you care.

You get the Red Cross cart filled with clothing, reading material and snacks and go off to the hospital wards, starting with orthopaedics. You take a deep breath as you enter the ward. You know you are about to visit 30 to 40 recent ... amputees.

At the first room a family is visiting their soldier and a little girl is rubbing an amputated leg. She looks up and says, "He is still my daddy".

At the next room an amputee tells you he just wants to be treated like a whole person when he returns home.

The next soldier shows you the Purple Heart that was pinned on him by President Bush.

In the next room the soldier tells you that when he saw the tourniquet go on his leg after his Humvee was hit by an IED he knew that his leg was gone.

During the day you meet many veterans from prior wars who are staying with their wounded sons.

In the hallway you see a soldier walking with his IV [intravenous fluid] pole. You thank him for his service, but he quickly responds, 'No need to thank me; I have the best job in the world.'

A soldier sits in a wheel chair at a computer. You casually ask if he is writing home. He says he is writing back to Iraq because he is worried about the men in his unit. They suffered 60 deaths and over 200 wounded during the war, the most of any unit in the war.

Your final mission of the day is to give an electric razor to a double arm amputee with new prostheses. You are amazed to see him reach up to take off his backpack, unzip it, take the razor from you, place it in the backpack, zip it up, and put it back on. You get the feeling that this young man is going to do just fine in the years ahead.

Your positive thoughts about the future of the men and women you have visited are reinforced when you see a double-leg amputee with his new prostheses pushing his wife in a wheel chair for exercise.

Sunday you go to church and thank God that America has young people like the ones you met at the hospital. You also pray that there will be no more wounded. But if there are, you ask for the strength to help them and their families.

In a visit to the WRAMC, the entertainer Cher witnessed for herself an aspect of the human cost of the wars in Iraq and Afghanistan:

The thing that I was most shocked by as I walked into the hospital was a boy about 19 or 20 years old who'd lost both of his arms. Everyone had lost either one arm, one limb or two limbs, or had lost one limb and there were a lot of legs that seemed to be missing and a couple of the boys told me it was because of their vehicles. The rockets pierce the vehicles so much it's like being kind of in a tin can. The walls of the Humvees are very soft and there's no protection. But three guys in the same vehicle had lost legs. And another thing that I saw was that if they'd lost one leg, that shrapnel had hit the other leg [it was] so devastating that they were having to pull the thigh to try to make the leg workable, but in some cases these boys had lost one leg, and the other leg was so damaged that they weren't sure what they were gonna be able to do.

A NEW OLD DISEASE

An old concept of 'pain as a disease in its own right' has recently resurfaced in the American magazine *Newsweek*. It suggested that chronic pain has to be addressed as a specific entity by using the high-tech tools of pain-clinic 'gurus' who believe that they are now better informed by new 'brain science'.

Chester Buckenmaier, a 'pain tsar' at WRAMC, a chief of pain medicine from Philadelphia and a director of the American Pain Foundation are investigating newly discovered pain receptors. They hope that they might explain the continuing physical pain that afflicts one in every five American war veterans, just as it does civilians. Their bold research and theories lead them into the 'parallel universe' of complementary and alternative medicine.

The idea is that, even on the battlefield, the sooner injured troops get access to the standard of pain relief used in civilian hospitals, the sooner they can break the noxious 'pain pathways' that may persist into later life. While we await details of their ground-breaking research, there is a 'takeaway' message in the *Newsweek* article that the time-honoured principles of using pain-relief narcotics such as morphine, administered by various routes and in various doses and frequencies, might have been inadequate, inappropriate or incorrect.

How revolutionary the techniques pioneered by Buckenmaier and his team prove to be will only be demonstrated by evidence-based, independent reports. In the meantime, the researchers are busily confronting the challenges of deciding what exactly is being treated and why the new treatments work, if they really do. Only time will tell how well they have understood the problems and how well they can manage them.

CHAPTER 23

'Middle' America

When the time comes for me, it will find me ready and standing tall. My life was not wasted and I died for what I believed in. I ask you to take comfort in that and do not mourn me, for now I wear my dress blues and stand guard at the gates of heaven. If there is only one thing you could do for me, do not let my nieces and nephews forget about me; let them know I loved them and I pray my sacrifice to them will be all they will ever have to pay for happiness in life.

– Letter written by a 23-year-old US Marine to a friend on 18 September 2001.[1]

Geoff Elliott's 2006 story 'Broken Heartland' in the *Weekend Australian Magazine* begins with the statement that, 'Support for Bush's war in Iraq is ebbing in Middle America where small communities bear the heaviest burden of grief.' It refers to the state of Wisconsin, but Middle America also comprises Illinois, Indiana, Iowa, Kansas, Michigan, Minnesota, Missouri, Nebraska, North and South Dakota and Ohio.

How to interpret Elliott's statement depends somewhat on definitions. Middle America is an imprecise term applied either to Central America or to the conservative, middle-class 'Mid-West' of the USA. Given the mixed geography and demography of Middle America, it is probably true that most US armed forces and casualties in war come from areas where, according to Elliott:

> ... the population has been static for the best part of a decade, jobs have been hard to come by, civil government is a big employer, and one of the options for jobs is for young people to join the military; it's the youth of Middle America who are carrying the burden of fighting in Iraq.

Modern American armed forces recruits are enlisted from blacks (who were over-represented), whites and Hispanics from middle-class backgrounds, with

---

1. The Marine died in a helicopter crash in Baghdad on 19 May 2003, the first Wisconsin native soldier to die in Iraq. In June 2006, his father said: 'Cut and run? I'd hate to see all the lives lost be wasted.'

moderate levels of education. Many of them volunteer out of patriotism or an inherited tradition. Others come from a supposed underclass of disadvantaged individuals looking for personal improvement by adopting an army life. Most probably get some of what they seek. Obviously, they accept the risks of injury and death, but many of them enlist for service more than once. Clearly, most wars involving the USA could not continue without the reliable contribution of the youth of Middle America.

An arbitrary definition of Middle America may be convenient in terms of socio-economic, racial and demographic factors, but the frequency-distribution of war casualties is no longer as clearly demarcated as in 2006. Subtle changes must be apparent to surgical teams if only in terms of repatriating the disabled to communities where rehabilitation and counselling services may vary in quality between locations, if not between states. Various statistical sources (including a report by Eric Ostermeyer of Smart Politics in August 2009) indicate that, while Southern states supply the largest number of military *recruits*, the Mid-Western area has had larger numbers of *casualties* per head of population.

It is not clear why such differences occur, but the 2008 US Census Bureau per capita death and injury rates showed that, *in raw numbers*, most casualties occurred in the Southern states (presumably with higher coloured numbers), followed by the West and Mid-West and then by the North-East. But the *per capita* casualty rates were highest in the Mid-West. Clearly, the less privileged of all communities must be more tempted to enlist than others. Whether they are subjected to the riskier assignments cannot be measured. For surgeons, no such discrimination would be expected or has ever been reported to have occurred or been complained of by troops of any ethnic groups.

While otherwise similar towns may vary in their political choices for no discernible reason, many parents, even some who have lost children in Iraq, believe that the job still has to be finished. There remains a strong feeling in humble parts of the Mid-West that it is 'not right to cut and run and ignore the lessons of Vietnam. We owe it to [those] who have died to finish the job.'

Many members of surgical teams working in Iraq must understand and share those views. If not, why are they there? Just to accelerate their surgical experience? Maybe so. After all, there could be no better and faster way of learning surgery, as Hippocrates observed more than 2,000 years ago, but surgeons' reasons to re-enlist seem to differ and change. There are older men who served in Vietnam and re-entered the surgical fray in Iraq or Afghanistan who may also feel a dedication to 'finishing the job'. Besides, nearly 70 per cent of all those treated by the Coalition in Iraq are local Iraqi civilians who could never get the superb standard of care that the Allied forces offer without discrimination or cost to patients.

Elliott's observations suggest that, regardless of the appalling stories and images that appear daily in the media, there is a substantial number of Americans and others who are not yet quite ready to dump Iraq and Afghanistan. Perhaps they sense that persistence just might win a prize they will one day consider worth the awful costs. High on the list of those willing to persist are doctors and nurses and other health professionals who yearn to contribute in something more rewarding than civilian life could ever offer them.

The predominant and intractable issues preventing peace in Iraq seem to be inter-ethnic, sectarian conflict and 'professional' insurgency, much of it imported. Nobody can be sure how the withdrawal of Allied forces will affect those factions, whether or not they are the direct concern of outsiders, medical or otherwise. One Iraqi surgeon, who will remain a target for kidnapping and assassination as long as he remains in Iraq, said that to avoid a 'disaster-zone' developing, '... not one in 20 million Iraqis really wants the Americans gone'. If the Americans do leave, doctors like him and his colleagues will flee to Jordan, Syria and other neighbouring states, worsening Iraq's medical problems.

Some families in Wisconsin complain that too few television cameras now await the plane-loads of wounded heroes airlifted back to the USA, destined for the over-burdened wards of Walter Reed and other army medical centres. As the war has progressed, these families have noticed fewer media pictures of troops undergoing physical rehabilitation or of families praying for news of loved ones. They have begun to think that the men injured in Iraq and Afghanistan may have become a 'new-disappeared' and that the media has lost interest in Middle America. The long haul of war may have become too ugly and unrewarding as more spectacular issues vie for media attention, but families thank God that surgical teams have not shared that loss of interest.

How US military personnel and their families interpret their President's acceptance of a Nobel Peace Prize while simultaneously committing 30,000 more troops to the Afghanistan conflict can only be imagined. No doubt, regardless of their origins, their pride, loyalty, national respect and future expectations of employment and status will provide some reward for placing their lives and limbs at risk.

Epilogue

A Dedication to Heroes
For every hundred men you send,
Ten should not even be here.
Eighty are nothing but targets.
Nine of them are real fighters.
We are lucky to have them; they the battle make.
Ah, but the one – one of them is a warrior.
And he will bring the others back.

– Heraclitus, Greek philosopher, 500 BC

AUSTRALIAN SURGEONS IN CAPTIVITY

Proudly We Served (revised by Vince Egan), a history of 2/5 Australian General Hospital in the Second World War, relates how some 170 members of the hospital volunteered to remain as POWs in Greece, Poland and Germany to look after the Australian wounded. The Germans treated them very well and left them unmolested to carry on their fine work.

Dr Rosalind Hearder records that 106 Australian doctors were prisoners of the Japanese during the Pacific War, forty-four of them on the infamous Burma–Thai Railway. Despite being cared for by their own doctors, one-third of all Australian prisoners held by the Japanese died in captivity. Among the many surgeons who cared for the Australians and others on the railway were Dr Edward Dunlop and Dr Albert Coates. They displayed great dedication and skill, often at the risk of retaliation from the Japanese; their contributions are universally acknowledged.

There were many other allied medical staff who cared selflessly for their mates and whose reputations have also become part of surgical history. One of them was Dr Kevin Fagan who was captured in Malaya in 1942. His manner and medical exploits give him an everlasting place in our medical history. Russell Braddon, a prisoner in Changi, described Fagan in his book, *The Naked Island*:

Above all there was the extraordinary courage and gentleness, and the incredible endurance of [Fagan]. Not only did he treat any man needing treatment to the best of his ability; he also carried men who fell. He carried the kit of men in danger of falling and he marched up and down the whole length of the column throughout its entire progress. If we marched 100 miles through the jungle, Kevin Fagan marched 200 miles and, when at the end of our night's trip, we collapsed and slept, he was there to clean blisters, set broken bones and render first aid. And all of it he did with the courtesy of a society specialist who is being richly paid for his attention and the ready humour of a man who is not tired at all ... he is [one of] the most inspiring men I have ever met. Some 20,000 British and Australian troops share my view.

In 2005, as a national gesture of gratitude for their sacrifices and slavery, the Australian government paid each POW of the Japanese, or surviving next of kin, the sum of $25,000.

Acronyms

AIF – Australian Imperial Force
ANZ – Australia and New Zealand
AWL – Absentee Without Leave
CPD – Citrate Potassium Dextrose
CSH – Combat Support Hospital
DC – District of Columbia
DVT – Deep Vein Thrombosis
ETO – European Theatre of Operations
FST – Forward Surgical Team
Humvee – High-mobility multi-purpose wheeled vehicle
ICRC – International Committee of the Red Cross
IED – Improvised Explosive Device
IRC – International Red Cross
JEMS – Journal of Emergency Medicine Society
LST – Landing Craft Tank
MASH – Mobile Army Surgical Hospital
MRAP – Mine-Resistant, Ambush-Protected Vehicle
MSF – Médecins Sans Frontières
NYDN – Not Yet Diagnosed Nervousness
NZPFOCA – New Zealand Permanent Force Old Comrades Association
POW – Prisoner of War
PTSD – Post Traumatic Stress Disorder
RMO – Australian Regimental Medical Officer
RPG – Rocket-Propelled Grenade
Serum – in blood banks, this refers to plasma with the white cells removed
SSTP – Surgical Shock Trauma Platoon
UNICEF – United Nations International Children's Emergency Fund
UNSW – University of New South Wales
USNS – United States Nursing Ship
USS – United States Ship
WRAMC – Walter Reed Army Medical Center
WRANS – Women's Royal Australian Naval Service

References

Chapter 1: Evolution of War Surgery

Anderson, K. D. 'Presidential Address,' *Bull. Am. Coll. Surg.* (2005)
Asimov, I. 'Hippocrates,' *Biol. Encycl. of Science and Technology* (Second Edition) (1982)
Battlefield Surgery 101: From the Civil War to Vietnam (National Museum of Health and Medicine Exhibit, Walter Reed Army Medical Center, 2005)
Breasted, J. *Edwin Smith Surgical Papyrus* (Chicago University Press, 1930)
Brehier, L. 'The Crusades', *Catholic Encyclopedia* (Appleton, 1908)
Brewer, C. *The Death of Kings (Richard I)* (Abson Books, 2000)
Burgh, J. *General Reflections on Standing Armies in Free Countries in Times of Peace* (The [US] Founders' Constitution, 1774)
Carlyon, L. *The Great War* (Macmillan, 2006)
Coates, J. B. Jr (editor in chief), *Surgery in World War II, Activities of Surgical Consultants, Vols I & II* (Medical Department, United States Army, Office of the Surgeon General, Washington DC, 1962 & 1964)
Connelly, O. *Blundering to Glory: Napoleon's Military Campaigns* (Third Edition) (Google Books, 2006)
Coupland, R. *War Wounds of Limbs; Surgical Management* (Butterworth Heinemann, 1993)
Crumplin, M. *Men of Steel: Surgery in Napoleonic Wars* (Quiller Press, 2007)
Crumplin, M. 'Surgery in the Napoleonic Wars.' Myles Gibson Military Lectures, *J. Roy. Coll. Surg.* (2002)
DeBakey, M. E. Personal communication (2007)
Dew, H. 'Chemotherapy in War Surgery,' *ANZ. J. Surg.* X (1940)
Drucker, C. 'Ambrose Pare and the Birth of the Gentle Art of Surgery,' *Yale J. Biol. Med.* 81 (2008)
Echols, M. ACW medical and surgical antiques (current and agreed reference)
Ellis, H. 'The Thomas Splint,' *J. Periop. Practice* (2007)
Evans, B. *Combat-Wise Platoon Sergeants* (36th Infantry Division Association, 26 May 1944)
Fisher, R. *Joseph Lister* (Stein and Day, 1977)
Geison, G. *The Private Science of Louis Pasteur* (Princeton University Press, 1995)
Gordon, R. *The Alarming History of Medicine* (Mandarin, 1993)
Gray, R. *War Wounds: Basic Surgical Management* (I.C.R.C., 1994)
Grigsby, B. 'The Social Position of the Surgeon in London, 1350–1450,' *Essays in Medieval Studies* (1996)
Grogono, B. 'Changing the hideous face of war,' *Brit. Med. J.* (1991)
Hawley, P. *And That Men Might Live! – The Story of the Medical Services, European Theatre of Operations* (Stars and Stripes, 1944–1945)
Holmes, R. (editor) *The Oxford Companion to Military History* (Oxford University Press, 2001)
Hume, E. *Victories of Army Medicine* (Lippincott Williams & Wilkins, 1943)
Hyer, R. 'Battlefield Protocols May Move to Civilian World,' *Medscape Medical News* (11 October, 2006)

Keegan, J. *The Face of War* (Penguin, 1978)

Keegan, J. *A History of Warfare* (Vintage, 1994)

Keegan, J. 'Perspective on Iraq,' *London Telegraph* (5 June 2004)

Kothare, S. 'Surgery in Ancient and Medieval Times,' *St John's Medical College J. Med.,* Bangalore (1991)

Le Carré, J. *The Honourable Schoolboy* (Hodder and Stoughton, 1977)

Lepage, J. D. *Medieval Armies and Weapons in Western Europe* (McFarland and Co., 2005)

Mitchell, P. *Medicine in the Crusades: Warfare, Wounds and the Medieval Surgeon* (Cambridge University Press, 2004)

Mitchiner, P. and Cowell, P. *Medical Organisation and Surgical Practice in Air Raids* (Churchill, 1939)

Nessen, S., Lounsbury. E. and Hetz, S. (editors) *War Surgery in Afghanistan and Iraq: A Series of Cases, 2003–2007* (Borden Institute, US Army, 2008)

Neuhaus, S. 'Post Vietnam – three decades of Australian military surgery,' *ADF Health J.,* Vol. 5 (April 2004)

Nobel Lectures 1901–1921, Physiology or Medicine, *Robert Koch* (Elsevier, 1961)

Oppenheimer, M. *All Work No Pay, Australian Civil Volunteers in War* (Ohio Productions, 2002)

Ortiz, J. 'The Revolutionary Flying Ambulance of Napoleon's Surgeon,' *U.S. Army Medical Department Journal* (Oct/Dec1998)

Pollard, A. 'Geoffrey Chaucer,' *Encycl. Britannica Vol. VI* (Cambridge University Press, 1910)

Russell, R., Williams, N. and Bulstrode, C. (editors) *Bailey & Love's Short Practice of Surgery* (twenty-third edition) (Arnold, 2000)

Sienfelder, L. *Semmelweis, I.* New York: *Catholic Encyclopedia* (Appleton, 1911)

Sequin, M. *Gallipoli: The Medical War* (UNSW Press, 1993)

Seward, D. *The Hundred Years War: The English in France, Agincourt* (Penguin, 1999)

Sheehan, P. 'Fixation with Appearances Turns Ugly,' *Sydney Morning Herald* (1 May 2006)

Steele, R. 'Religion and Medicine,' *Med. J. Aust* (20 September 1969)

Stinger, Col. H. 'Operation Iraqi Freedom,' *Bull. Am. Coll. Surg.* (3 March 2004)

Sunshine, J. 'Function of a Field Hospital during WWII,' *Providence (RI) Sunday Journal* (1994)

Takrouri, M. *Ancient Surgery and Anaesthesia Practice in Arabic Countries* (King Khalid University Hospital, 2002)

Takrouri, M. 'Surgery 700 Years Ago,' *Saudi Newsletter* (2002)

Taylor, F. O. *Memoirs and Diaries* (Everyman at War, 1918)

US Army Medical Department, Surgical Consultants, World War 2, Vols 1 & 2

Vertrees, A., Kellicut, D., Ottman, S., Peoples, G. and Shriner, C. 'Early Definitive Abdominal Closure Using Serial Closure Technique – Afghanistan and Iraq,' *J. Am. Coll. Surg.* (May 2006)

Vertrees, A., Kellicut, D., Ottman, S., Peoples, G. and Shriner, C. 'Modern Management of Complex Open Abdominal Wounds of War: a 5-Year Experience,' *J. Am. Coll. Surg.* (December 2008)

Welling, D., Burns, D. and Rich, N. 'Delayed Recognition – Larrey and Les Invalides,' *J. Am. Coll. Surg.* (2005)

Whayne, T. and DeBakey, M. E. *Cold Injury – Ground Type* (US Army Medical Department, 1958)

Chapter 2: Surgery Comes of Age with Anaesthesia

ANZ. J. Surg., [Various authors and dates]: Ackland, T. H., Clarke, B., Dew, H., Gray, R., Grogan, R., Hurley, T., King, E., Lesley, D., Nichols, P., Poate, H., Rank, B., Renou, C., Rogers, L., Somerset, J., Wakefield, A., Yeates, D. and Yeates, J.

Barr, M. *Surgery, Sand and Saigon Tea.* (Allen & Unwin, 2001)

Bodemer, C. 'Baron Dominique-Jean Larrey, Napoleon's Surgeon,' *Bull. Am. Coll. Surg.,* 67 (1982)

DeBakey, M. E. Personal communication (2007)

Gawande, A. 'Casualties of War, Military Care for the Wounded from Iraq and Afghanistan,' *N. Eng. J. Med.* 2004, Vol. 351: 2471–5

Gordon, R. *The Alarming History of Medicine* (Mandarin, 1993)

Holmes, R. (editor) *The Oxford Companion to Military History* (Oxford University Press, 2001)

Kaufman, M. *Robert Liston: Surgery's Hero* (RCS Edin., 2009)

Koefod, J. Personal communication (2006)

Magee, R. 'Amputation Through the Ages: The Oldest Major Surgical Operation.' *ANZ. J. Surg.* 68 (1998)

Mitchell, P. *Medicine in the Crusades: Warfare, Wounds and the Medieval Surgeon* (Cambridge University Press, 2004)

Morrison, C. 'A Military Surgeon Questions the Value of a Forward Austere Surgical Team,' *J. Am. Coll. Surg.* (August 2006)

Ortiz, J. 'The Revolutionary Flying Ambulance of Napoleon's Surgeon,' *U.S. Army Medical Department Journal* (Oct/Dec 1998)

Perry, C. 'Life and Death Every Day for Iraq Medics and Doctors in Iraq,' CNN (10 May 2006)

'Reed Elsevier and the International Arms Trade,' *The Lancet* (10–15 September, 2005)

Sequin, M. *Gallipoli: The Medical War* (UNSW Press, 1993)

'The New War on Pain,' *Newsweek* (4 June 2007)

Chapter 3: The Special Challenges of Military Medicine

Annan, K. *We the Peoples* – Report to UN General Assembly (October 2000)

Bruce, A. *An Illustrated Companion to the First World War* (Michael Joseph Ltd, 2002)

Champion, H., Mabee, M., Meredith, J. 'The State of US Trauma Systems,' *J. Am. Coll. Surg.,* 203 (2006)

Committee on Trauma. 'Disasters from Biological and Chemical Terrorism,' *J. Am. Coll. Surg.* (2001)

DeBakey, M. E. Personal communication (2007)

Editors, 'International Arms Fair,' *The Lancet* (September 2005)

Elliott, G. 'Broken Heartland,' *Weekend Australian Magazine* (25–26 June 2006)

Eisenhower, D. Speech [on weapons] before American Society of Newspaper Editors (April 16, 1953)

Gawande, A. 'Casualties of War, Military Care for the Wounded from Iraq and Afghanistan,' *N. Eng. J. Med.* 2004, 351: 2471–5

Gibbins, J. Personal communication (2006)

Global Security. *Notes on Casualties in Iraq* (June 2008)

Gordon, R. *The Alarming History of Medicine* (Mandarin, 1993)

Hoge, C. 'Mild Head Injury Not a Main Driver of Posttraumatic Stress Disorder in Soldiers,' *N. Eng. J. Med.* (January 2008)

'International Arms Fair,' *The Lancet* Vol. 366: 868 (2005)

Khat, A. 'Revenge Killings Take Toll,' *The Weekend Australian* (30 September 2006)

Kick, R. *U.S. Military Personnel Wounded in Iraq and Afghanistan* (The Memory Hole, 2003)

Kirk, N. *Prevention of Loss of Manpower from Psychic Disorders* – US Surgeon General's Report (April 1944)

Koefod, J. Personal communication (1985–2006)

Magee, R. 'Muskets, Musket Balls and the Wounds they Made,' *ANZ. J. Surg.* 1995, 65: 890–5

McKnight, G. *Breach of Trust: How the Warren Commission Failed the Nation and Why* (University of Kansas Press, 2005)

Murji, A., Gomez, M., Knighton, J. and Fish, J. 'Emotional Implications of Working in a Burn Unit,' *J. Burn Care & Research* (Jan/Feb 2006)

Nelson, J. 'When Doctors go to War,' *New. Eng. J. Med.* (6 January 2005)

'The New War on Pain', *Newsweek* (4 June 2007)

Ruggenberg, R. *The Heritage of the Great War (1914–1918)* (2007)

Steward, H. D. *Recollections of a Regimental Medical Officer* (Melbourne University Press, 1983)

'US soldier acquitted in Iraq "fragging" case,' ABC News Online (December 2008)

Zoroyo, G. 'Doctors' Dilemmas in Iraq,' *USA Today* (6 May 2006)

Zoroya, G. 'Pentagon Holds Brain Injury Data,' *USA Today* (6 August 2006)

Chapter 4: Gunpowder and its Progeny

Gordon, R. *The Alarming History of Medicine* (Mandarin, 1993)

McGrory, D., Evans, M. 'Hunt for the Master of Explosives,' *The Times* (13 July 2005)

Nessen, S., Lounsbury. E. and Hetz, S. (editors) *War Surgery in Afghanistan and Iraq: A Series of Cases, 2003–2007* (Borden Institute, US Army, 2008)

Ruffell, W. *The Gun – Gunpowder* (NZPFOCA, September 1992)

Ruggenberg, R. *The Heritage of the Great War (1914–1918)* (2007)

Sheehan, P. 'Fixation with Appearances Turns Ugly,' *Sydney Morning Herald* (1 May 2006)

Shuck, H., Sohlman, R. *The Life of Alfred Nobel* (Heineman, 1929)

Chapter 5: Body-Armour

Peleg, K. 'Does body-armor protect from firearm injuries?' *J. Am. Coll. Surg.* (2005)

Chapter 6: Crimean War Catastrophe

Dunant, H. *A Memory of Solferino* (ICRC, 1986)

Holmes, R. (editor) *The Oxford Companion to Military History* (Oxford University Press, 2001)

McCoubrey, H. 'Before Geneva Law; A British Surgeon in the Crimean War,' *International Review of the Red Cross* (Cambridge University Press, Jan/Feb 1995)

Sweetman, J. 'The Crimean War,' *Br. Med. J.*, 2 (1899)

Wrench, E. 'Lessons of the Crimean War,' *Br. Med. J.*, 2, (1899)

Chapter 7: American Civil War – The Dawn of Modern Surgery

Bean, W. *Walter Reed: A Biography* (University of Virginia Press, 1982)

Encyclopaedia of the Civil War (The Civil War Society, 2002)

Floyd, B. *Medicine in the Civil War* (Toledo University Library, 1995)

Goelinitz, J. *Civil War Medicine: An Overview* (Department History, Ohio State University, 2005)

Heidler, D. 'The American Civil War: A Political, Social and Medical History,' *Encyclopedia of ACW* (2002)

Holmes, R. (editor) *The Oxford Companion to Military History* (Oxford University Press, 2001)

Hume, E. *Victories of Army Medicine* (Lippincott, 1943)

McWhorter, P. *Civil War Medicine* (Son of the South, 2006)

Musto, R. 'Treatment of the Wounded at Gettysburg: Jonathan Letterman. The Father of Modern Battlefield Medicine,' *Gettysburg Magazine,* Issue 37 (2007)

Nofi, A. *A Civil War Treasury* (Da Capo Press, 1995)

Perrett, B. *Last Stand: Famous Battles Against the Odds* (Arms and Armour, 1993)

Chapter 8: War Against Politicians

Brown, D. 'Four Score and Seven Ways to Save Abe,' *Sydney Morning Herald* (26 May 2007)

'Robert Kennedy Assassination: Revisions and Rewrites' (Courtroom Television Network LLC, 2005)

'Essential JFK Assassination,' *Trivia*, Vol. 2 (1965)

Melanson, P. *Who Killed Robert Kennedy?* (Odonian Press, 1993)

Sloffer, C. and Hanigan, W. 'A gunshot wound to the cervical spine: The case of the Presidential assassin,' *Bull. Am. Coll. Surg.* (January 2007)

Trunkey, D. and Farjah, F. 'Medical and surgical care of our four assassinated Presidents,' *J. Am. Coll. Surg.* (2005)

Chapter 9: The First World War, 1914–1918

Arthur, G. *Life of Lord Kitchener* (Macmillan, 1920)

Coates, J. B. Jr (editor in chief) *Surgery in World War II, Activities of Surgical Consultants, Vols I & II* (Medical Department, United States Army, Office of the Surgeon General, Washington DC, 1962 & 1964)

Dew, H. 'Chemotherapy in War Surgery,' *ANZ. J. Surg.* X (1940)

Dolev, E. *Allenby's Military Medicine: Life and Death in WWI Palestine* (Tauris & Co., 2007)

Eisenstadt, D. *The British Mandate: Jerusalem.* (Ingeborg Rennert Center, May 1997)

Gardner, D. *Surgeon, Scientist, Soldier: The Life and Times of Henry Wade.* (The Royal Society of Medicine Press, 2005)

Hartley, P. *The Gallipoli Front* (King College, London, Project façade, 2005)

Hayward, J. *Memoirs & Diaries: A Casualty Clearing Station* (First World War Com., 2 October 2001)

Holmes, R. (editor) *The Oxford Companion to Military History* (Oxford University Press, 2001)

Keegan, J. *The Face of War* (Penguin, 1978)

Keegan, J. *A History of Warfare* (Vintage, 1994)

Keegan, J. 'Perspective on Iraq,' *London Telegraph* (5 June 2004)

Kennedy, S. 'WWI soldiers cleared of cowardice,' ABC Online Australia (17 August 2006)

Kirkup, J. 'Fracture Care of Friend and Foe during World War I,' *ANZ. J. Surg.* 2003, 73: 453–59

Mitchiner, P. and Cowell, P. *Medical Organisation and Surgical Practice in Air Raids* (Churchill, 1939)

Ruggenberg, R. *The Heritage of the Great War (1914–1918)* (2007)

Serle, G. *John Monash: A Biography* (MUP, 1982)

Smith, H. *Memoirs of an Ambulance Company Officer, St Mihiel* (Doomsday, 1940)

Tyquin, M. *Gallipoli: The Medical War* (UNSW Press, 1993)

Tyquin, M. *Little by Little* (Australian Military History Publications, 2003)

Chapter 10: Infections, Antiseptics and Antibiotics

Gordon, R. *The Alarming History of Medicine* (Mandarin, 1993)

Henderson, J. 'The yellow brick road to penicillin: a story of serendipity,' *Mayo Clin. Proc.* Vol. 72 (1997)

Hyams, K., Wignall, F., Escamilla, J. and Oldfield, E. 'The impact of infectious diseases on the health of U.S. troops – Desert Shield and Desert Storm,' *Clin. Infect. Dis.* Washington DC, 1995, 20: 1497–1504

Macfarlane, G. *Howard Florey* (Oxford University Press, 1979)

Chapter 11: Red Gold

Nessen, S., Lounsbury. E. and Hetz, S. (editors) *War Surgery in Afghanistan and Iraq: A Series of Cases, 2003-2007* (Borden Institute, US Army, 2008)

Pelis, K. 'Edward Archibald's notes on blood transfusion in war surgery,' *Wilderness and Environmental Medicine* Vol. 13, No. 3 (2002)

Chapter 12: The Second World War, 1939–1945

Andrews, L. *No Time for Romance* (Harrap, 1977)

'Aussies at Tobruk,' *War and Game* (24 February 2008)

Bell, R. *Casualty clearance – the WWII nurses regiment*, Anzac Day Commemoration Committee (1 November 2007)

Coates, J. B. Jr (editor in chief), *Surgery in World War II, Activities of Surgical Consultants, Vols I & II* (Medical Department, United States Army, Office of the Surgeon General, Washington DC, 1962 & 1964)

Cohen, E. *The Mystique of U.S. Air Power* (US Council on Foreign Relations, 1994)

Consultants, Vols I & II (Medical Department, United States Army, Office of the Surgeon General, Washington DC, 1962 & 1964)

De Vries, S. *Heroic Women in War: Tales of Bravery from Gallipoli to Kokoda* (HarperCollins, 2007)

De Vries, S. *To Hell and Back: The Banned Story of Gallipoli* (HarperCollins, 2004)

Egan, V. *Proudly We Served – 2/5 AGH* (Australian Military History Publications, revised 2007)

Gentile, A. *World War II Combat Medic. 84th Infantry Division, WWII* (2003)

Goodman, R. *A Hospital at War* (Boolarong, 1983)

Grogan, R. 'The operation of forward surgical teams in the Kokoda-Buna Campaigns,' *ANZ. J. Surg.* 1998, 68: 68–73

Holmes, R. (editor) *The Oxford Companion to Military History* (Oxford University Press, 2001)

Howden, S. 'Courage under fire of pioneer city surgeon (Henry Wade),' *Scotsman Evening News* (11 November 2005)

'In Memoriam: Major General Paul R Hawley,' *Ann. R. Coll. Surg. Engl.*, 38 1966

Jeppeson, J. *Constant care, the RAN Health Services, 1915* (Australian Military History Publications, 2002)

King, E. 'Surgery in the desert,' *ANZ. J. Surg.* XI (1941)

MacDonald, C. *A Time for Trumpets: The Untold story of the Battle of the Bulge* (Bantam, 1984)

Moseley, L. *Faces from the Fire. The Biography of Sir Archibald McIndoe* (Weidenfeld and Nicholson, 1962)

Not only a Hero: The Donkey, Anzac Day Commemoration Committee (1998)

Plunkett, G. *Chemical Warfare in Australia* (Australian Military History Publications, 2007)

Spurling, R. and Woodhall, B. (editors) *Surgery in WWII – Neurosurgery*, Vol. 1 (Medical Department, US Army, 1958)

Steinert, D. *The History of WWII Medicine* (WWII Combat Medic, 5 April 2002)

Steward, H. *Recollections of a Regimental Medical Officer* (Melbourne University Press, 1983)

Sunshine, J. 'Function of a Field Hospital during WWII,' *Providence (RI) Sunday Journal* (1994)

Sunshine, J. Personal communication (2007-2010)

Tavernise, S. 'At least 600,000 civilians killed in Iraq, studies find,' *Sydney Morning Herald* (12 October 2006)

Taylor, F. W. 'Gunshot Wounds of the Abdomen,' *Ann. Surg.* (February 1973)

The Nurses' Experience of Gallipoli from their Letters (various quoted authors) (Australian Department Veterans' Affairs, 2007)

Whayne, T. and DeBakey, M. E. *Cold Injury – Ground Type* (US Army Medical Department, 1958)
Williamson, B. *I Remember General Patton's Principles* (Quotation, 1984)

Chapter 13: Nuremberg and Other Agonies

Andrus, B. *The Infamous of Nuremberg* (Leslie Frewin, 1969)
Taylor, T. (prosecutor) *Trials of War Criminals, Nuremberg Military Tribunals (1946–1949)*. Washington DC, USA, 1949–1953

Chapter 14: 'Small' Wars

Bolton, R. 'The Media Report reflects on the Vietnam War,' ABC Radio National (3 June 1999)
'Committee on Gulf War Veterans' Illnesses' (ABC News online, November 2008)
Cowdrey, A. (editor) *U.S. Army in the Korean War: The Medics' War* (US Army Center Military History, 1987)
Cushman, J., Patchter, H. and Beaton, H. 'Two New York City Hospitals, Surgical Response to the 11 September 2001,' *J. Trauma, Infection, and Critical Care,* 54 (January 2003)
'From our Correspondents: 11 September 2001,' *The New Yorker* (24 September 2001)
Goldberg, J. 'Behind Mubarak,' *The New Yorker* (8 October 2001)
Grauwin, P. *Doctor at Dien-Bien-Phu* (Harrison, 1955)
Korean War: Early Defeat, Turning the Tide, China Enters War, Stalemate, Civilian Casualties, Aftermath. California Pacific Tours (October 2009)
Maxwell, A. F. B. *Korean War, 1950–1953* (Air University Library, 1996)
McCallion, T. and Heightman, A. 'Lessons Learned from 9/11,' *J.E.M.S.,* Vol. 31, (1 September 2006)
McLeod, S. 'Bougainville: departure of Australian police,' ABC Online (17 May 2005)
Médecins sans Frontières. *Voices from the Field* (MSF Australia, 2005)
Memorandum of Understanding to Protect Children's Rights. UNICEF and Liberia's Ministry of National Defence, Monrovia, Liberia (2 December 2009)
Meyerowitz, J. 'Looking South,' *The New Yorker* (24 September 2001)
New York Downtown Hospital, *Response to September 11, 2001* (2005)
NewYork-Presbyterian Hospital/Weill Cornell Medical. 'Learning from 9/11,' *Medical News Today* (11 September 2008)
Plunkett, G. *Chemical Warfare in Australia* (Australian Military History Publications, 2007)
Roccaforte, J. D. *The World Trade Center Attack*. The Critical Care Forum, New York (6 November 2001)
Sasaki, C. 'Holding death at bay in Vietnam,' *Vietnam Magazine* (21 April 2006)
Skinner, A. 'War in Congo,' *Nation & World* (27 September 2002)
Spragg, G. *When Good Men do Nothing* (Australian Military History Publications, 2003)
'The Talk of the Town: Today and After,' *The New Yorker* (24 September 2001)
Thompson, G. 'In Haiti, Politics and Gunfire Engulf UN Force,' *New York Times* (24 January 2006)

Chapter 15 Iraq and Afghanistan

'1800 die in Baghdad in July, morgue says,' ABC News Online (10 August 2006)
'Operating Under Fire,' ABC TV, Sydney (February 2007)
Al Sheibani, B., Hadi, N. and Hassoon, T. 'Iraq Lacks Facilities and Expertise in Emergency Medicine,' *B.M.J.* (21 October 2006)
Brown, A. 'Vascular Surgery Now Saving More Limbs After Battlefield Injuries,' Reuters (19 November 2007)

Brulliard, K. 'Learning from Saddam,' *Washington Post,* (5 May 2007)

Clouse, W., Rasmussen, T., Peck, M., Eliason, J., Cox, M., Bowser, A., Jenkin, D., Smith, D. and Rich N. 'In-theater management of vascular injury: Balad Vascular Registry,' *J. Am. Coll. Surg.* (April 2007)

Eastman A. 'Dispatch from Landstuhl,' *Bull. Am. Coll. Surg.* (December 2007)

Eccleston, R. 'The Thin Khaki Line,' *The Weekend Australian* (28–29 October 2006)

Goodwin, J. 'Behind the Scenes, Surgical Unit Treats Fallujah's Casualties,' *Marine Corps News* (7 December 2004)

Grant, D. 'Elsevier Ditches Arms Trade,' *The Scientist* (4 June 2007)

Hull, A. and Priest, D. 'The Hotel Aftermath,' *Washington Post* (19 February 2007)

Hyams, K. 'The Impact of Infectious Diseases on the Health of US troops – Desert Shield and Desert Storm,' *Clin. Infect. Dis.* 1995, 20: 1497–1504

Kennedy, S. *WW1 Soldiers Cleared of Cowardice* ABC Radio AM (17 August 2006)

Knudsen, M., Mitchell, F. and Johannigman, J. 'Landstuhl Regional Medical Center, Germany: Trauma Verification Review,' *Bull. Am. Coll. Surg.* (December 2007)

Liebl, V. 'An Interview with an Iraqi Soldier,' *Command Magazine* (Nov/Dec 1991)

Moulton, S. 'Iraq: Getting the Right Troops in the Right Places,' *International Herald Tribune* (16–17 September 2006)

Nelson, T., Wall, D., Stedje-Larsen, E., Clark, R., Chambers, L. and Bohman, H. 'Predictors of mortality in close proximity; blast injuries during Operation Iraqi Freedom,' *J. Am. Coll. Surg.* (2005)

Nessen, S., Lounsbury. E. and Hetz, S. (editors) *War Surgery in Afghanistan and Iraq: A Series of Cases, 2003–2007* (Borden Institute, US Army, 2008)

Neuhaus, S. 'Post Vietnam – Three Decades of Australian Military Surgery,' *ADF Health*, Vol. 5 (April 2004)

Pike, J. 'Notes on Casualties in Iraq,' *Global Security* (27 April 2005)

Post, T. (US Casualty, Iraq), Minnesota Public Radio (29 December 2004)

Renou, D. 'Early Treatment of Battle Casualties of Soft Tissue and Bone,' Presentation, R.A.C. Surgs. (15 May 1995)

Sharwood, P. 'Monday Morning in Downtown Balad,' Royal Australian Army, *Medical Corps Magazine* (2005)

Stengel, R. 'Osama bin Laden and the Idea of Progress,' *Time Magazine* (21 December 2001)

Stinger, Col. H. 'Operation Iraqi Freedom,' *Bull. Am. Coll. Surg.* (March 2004)

Sunshine, J. 'Function of a Field Hospital during WWII,' *Providence (RI) Sunday Journal* (1994)

Vick, K. 'Roadside Bombs Have Devastated Troops and Doctors Who Treat Them,' *Washington Post Foreign Service* (12 April 2004)

Zucchino, D. 'The Lifeline,' *Los Angeles Times* (2–3 April 2006)

Chapter 16: Women and War Injuries

McCall, S. *Lessons Learned by Army Nurses in Combat* (US Army War College, 1993)

Oppenheimer, M. 'Women missing in action – why has ANZAC become a "boys' only" story?' News Ltd, Sydney (7 November 2007)

Wilson, P. *Returned and Service Nurses Club of Victoria* (4 October 2006)

Chapter 17: The Human Costs of War

Sappenfield, M. 'Returning from War, Soldiers Splurge,' *Christian Science Monitor* (18 April 2006)

Tavernise, S. 'At Least 600,000 Civilians Killed in Iraq, Studies Find,' *Sydney Morning Herald* (12 October 2006)

Zebari, H. 'Iraq Fears US Troops will be Withdrawn,' *AAP,* (September 2008)

Zucchino, D. 'The Lifeline,' *Los Angeles Times* (2–3 April 2006)

Chapter 18: The Thieves of Minds and Men

Alexander, D. 'Early Mental Health Intervention after Disasters,' *Psychiatric Bulletin* (2005)

Dent, O., Richardson, B., Wilson, S., Goulston, K. and Murdoch, C. 'Postwar Mortality Among Australian World War II Prisoners of the Japanese,' *Med. J. Aust.* 150 (3 April 1989)

Gibbins, J. Personal communication (2006)

Holmes, R. (editor) *The Oxford Companion to Military History* (Oxford University Press, 2001)

Lambeth, L. Personal communication (2006)

Ruggenberg, R. *The Heritage of the Great War (1914–1918).* The Netherlands, 2007.

Rutherford, G. 'Long-Term Consequences of Traumatic Brain Injury,' *Gulf War and Health;* Vol. 7 (US Departments of Defence and Veterans' Affairs, 2008)

US Army Medical Department, Surgical Consultants, World War 2, Vols 1 & 2

'US Army Battles Rising Suicide Rate,' ABC News Online (1 February 2008)

Chapter 19: Bombs, Booby Traps and Land Mines

Eisler, P. and Morrison, B. 'Troops at Risk – IEDs in Iraq,' *USA Today* (16 July 2007)

Georgy, M. 'Vigilance Vital to Soldiers in Battle against Suicide Bombers,' *The Scotsman* (5 November 2004)

Nessen, S., Lounsbury. E. and Hetz, S. (editors) *War Surgery in Afghanistan and Iraq: A Series of Cases, 2003–2007* (Borden Institute, US Army, 2008)

US Army Medical Department, Surgical Consultants, World War 2, Vols 1 & 2

US Senate Subcommittee on Foreign Relations, *The Global Landmine Crisis* (May 3, 1994)

Chapter 20: The Arms Merchants

Croddy, E. *Chemical and Biological Warfare* (Copernicus Press, 2001)

Hartung, W. *Welfare for Arms Dealers: The Hidden Costs of the Arms Trade* (New York World Policy Institute, 1996)

'UK is world's biggest arms dealer [2007],' ABC News online (June 2008)

Chapter 21: The Faces of Terror

'Airline plot could have killed thousands,' ABC News Online (11 August 2006)

Almogy, G. and Rivkind, A. I. 'Surgical lessons learned from suicide bombing attacks,' *J. Am. Coll. Surg.* (2005)

Cushman, J., Patchter, H. and Beaton, H. 'Two New York City Hospitals,' Surgical 'Response to the 11 September 2001,' *J. Trauma, Infection, and Critical Care,* 54 (January 2003)

Dostoyevsky, F. *Notes from Underground.* Ch. 11 (1864)

From our Correspondents: 11 September 2001, *The New Yorker* (24 September 2001)

Goldberg, J. 'Behind Mubarak,' *The New Yorker* (8 October 2001)

Grant, D. 'Elsevier Ditches Arms Trade,' *The Scientist* (4 June 2007)

Grogono, B. 'Changing the Hideous Face of War,' *Brit. Med. J.* (1991)

Le Carré, J. 'Terrorism,' *The Times* (24 October 2001)

Lettieri, C. *Disaster Medicine: Understanding the Threat and Minimising the Effects.* Medscape Emergency Medicine, 2006; 1(1)

McCallion, T. and Heightman, A. 'Lessons Learned from 9/11,' *J.E.M.S.* 31 (1 September 2006)

McGrory, D. and Evans, M. 'Hunt for the Master of Explosives,' *The Times* (13 July 2005)

Meyerowitz, J. 'Looking South,' *The New Yorker* (24 September 2001)

Miller K. and Freinberg, T. 'Eye Witness Reports [London bombing],' London. Telegraph Media Group (10 July 2005)

Mitchiner, P. and Cowell, P. *Medical Organisation and Surgical Practice in Air Raids* (Churchill, 1939)

Nettnin, S. 'Emergency Life Support for Civilians in War Zones,' *Online journals* (3 November 2005)

New York Downtown Hospital. 'Response to September 11, 2001,' (2005)

New York-Presbyterian Hospital/Weill Cornell Medical. 'Learning from 9/11,' *Medical News Today* (11 September 2008)

Sheffy, N., Mintz, Y., Rivkind, A. and Shapira, S. 'Terror-related injuries: gunshot versus fragments,' *J. Am. Coll. Surg.* (September 2006)

Roccaforte, J. D. *The World Trade Center Attack*, The Critical Care Forum, New York (11 June 2001)

'The Talk of the Town: Today and After,' *The New Yorker* (24 September 2001)

'Twin bombings leave dozens dead,' ABC News Online (January 2007)

Chapter 22: Amputees – The Everlasting Army

American Legion Auxiliary Unit 270. *The Angels of Mercy: Volunteering at Walter Reed Medical Center* (2004)

Buckenmaier, C. 'The Changing Science of Pain,' *Newsweek* (Mary Carmichael) (4 June 2007)

Ellis, H. *A History of Surgery* (Greenwich, 2001)

Fox, C., Gillespie, D., Cox, E., Sumeru, G., Kragh J, Salinas, J. and Holcomb, J. *Strategy for Vascular Injury in a Combat Support Hospital: Case Control Study* (WRAMC, February 2008)

'History of War Surgery,' *Encyclopaedia Britannica Inc. On-line* (2006)

Magee, R. 'Amputation Through the Ages: The Oldest Major Surgical Operation,' *ANZ. J. Surg.* 68 (1998)

Nessen, S., Lounsbury. E. and Hetz, S. (editors) *War Surgery in Afghanistan and Iraq: A Series of Cases, 2003–2007* (Borden Institute, US Army, 2008)

'Volunteering at Walter Reed Medical Center,' *War Surgery* and *General Publications-Assistance* (21 April 2006)

Chapter 23: 'Middle' America

Sappenfield, M. 'Returning from War, Soldiers Splurge,' *Christian Science Monitor* (18 April 2006)

Epilogue

Hearder, R. 'Carers in captivity: Australian prisoners-of-war medical officers,' *Australian Government Defence Magazine* (2006)

Pezzutti, B, *Kevin Fagan, Surgeon, WW2*, Mention, NSW Parliament 9 September 1992, referring to *The Naked Island* by Russell Braddon

Smithhurst, B. A. 'Distinguished Australian Military Surgeons,' *ANZ. J. Surg.* 1989, 59: 731–741

Thomas, P. *Army Doctor – Reminiscences of an Australian Medical Officer WWII* (Pilpel & Co., 1981)

Note on the Author

Ten years after the atom bomb was dropped on Japan to end the Second World War, John Wright graduated from the University of Sydney with high honours and as a professorial resident at the Royal Prince Alfred Hospital. He was surgical superintendent of the hospital in 1960, with a Fellowship of the Royal Australasian College of Surgeons when he departed Sydney for overseas studies. By then he was totally besotted with the perilously fragile marriage of surgery and high technology – the basis of pioneering open-heart surgery.

After two years as Senior Surgical Registrar in Liverpool, England, he was appointed to the distinguished Stanford University in San Francisco; he gained the first Australian honorary fellowship of the twin American Colleges of Surgeons and Chest Physicians and was awarded senior membership of the American Society of Thoracic Surgeons. Those fabulous years at the top of the surgical world led to further experience at the University of Michigan before he returned to Sydney to become the first Australian to receive a professorial cardio-thoracic appointment. He worked in the University of New South Wales teaching hospitals for twenty-five years, during which time he was appointed Foundation Head of Paediatric Cardiac Surgery at the Prince of Wales Hospital, Sydney.

Dr Wright admits that cardio-thoracic surgery has been kinder to him than he ever expected; in his opinion it is by far the most brilliant of all specialities for its sheer innovation, technology and sense of adventure. His principles, taught to a dozen cardio-thoracic specialists throughout the world, include lifelong involvement in research, free care to the less privileged and constant collaboration with world leaders in the northern hemisphere. He has written and published hundreds of scientific articles, many showing how war surgery, heart surgery and trauma management tightly stretch the limits of medical science.

He believes his pre-occupation with frontier surgery arose from memories of his schooldays in the Second World War, when lives and families were destroyed, and from the modest courage of men he later met, who bravely attempted to conceal the everlasting scars of their wars. In them, he heard Winston Churchill's immortal words of 1941: 'Never give in. Never give in. Never, never, never, never – in nothing, great or small, large or petty – never give in ...' These words have never left Dr Wright's surgical mind.

John Wright MB, BS (Hons), FRACS, FACS, MSTS is the author of two surgical textbooks and over 200 peer-reviewed surgical articles.

Index